Praise for Jennifer Ashton and *Your Body Beautiful*

"The author's positive attitude, generally practical health recommendations and sassy style combine to lend her professional advice wide appeal." —*KIRKUS REVIEWS*

"Combination pep talk and warning, Ashton's message that women can and should take control of their own future health in these critical decades is backed up by current research and up-to-the-minute disease-prevention info." —*PUBLISHERS WEEKLY*

"Dr. Ashton helps women reclaim the most vibrant years of their lives by redefining women's health in the modern age. She will put a tiger in your tank." —DR. MEHMET OZ, host of *The Dr. Oz Show*

"Dr. Jennifer Ashton has provided a one-stop shop for all the tools we need to live the vibrant, healthy, and sexy life we all want and deserve." —DR. LAURA BERMAN, host of *In the Bedroom* on the OWN television network

"If you want to look and feel your best after forty (and who doesn't?), *Your Body Beautiful* is for you. Dr. Ashton offers groundbreaking tools that help you actually control the way you age. Follow these techniques, and this can be the healthiest, sexiest, most energized and beautiful stage of your entire life. This is the book all your girlfriends will be raving about—and for good reason." —KATHY SMITH, author of *Kathy Smith's Lift Weights to Lose Weight*

"Dr. Ashton has done a terrific job of creating a five-week program that any woman or mom can follow. The insight into our lives and the tools she provides will make an immediate and long-lasting change in anyone's life! I highly recommend it." — DARA TORRES, twelve-time Olympic medalist, motivational speaker, and mother

AVERY

a member of

Penguin Group (USA) Inc.

New York

YOUR BODY
BEAUTIFUL

Clockstopping Secrets
to Staying Healthy, Strong, and Sexy
in Your 30s, 40s, and Beyond

Jennifer Ashton, M.D.

with Christine Rojo

Published by the Penguin Group

Penguin Group (USA) Inc., 375 Hudson Street, New York, New York 10014, USA • Penguin Group (Canada), 90 Eglinton Avenue East, Suite 700, Toronto, Ontario M4P 2Y3, Canada (a division of Pearson Penguin Canada Inc.) • Penguin Books Ltd, 80 Strand, London WC2R 0RL, England • Penguin Ireland, 25 St Stephen's Green, Dublin 2, Ireland (a division of Penguin Books Ltd) • Penguin Group (Australia), 707 Collins Street, Melbourne, Victoria 3008, Australia (a division of Pearson Australia Group Pty Ltd) • Penguin Books India Pvt Ltd, 11 Community Centre, Panchsheel Park, New Delhi–110 017, India • Penguin Group (NZ), 67 Apollo Drive, Rosedale, Auckland 0632, New Zealand (a division of Pearson New Zealand Ltd) • Penguin Books Rosebank Office Park, 181 Jan Smuts Avenue, Parktown North 2193, South Africa • Penguin China, B7 Jaiming Center, 27 East Third Road North, Chaoyang District, Beijing 100020, China

Penguin Books Ltd, Registered Offices: 80 Strand, London WC2R 0RL, England

First Paperback edition 2012
Copyright © 2012 by Jennifer Ashton, M.D.

All rights reserved. No part of this book may be reproduced, scanned, or distributed in any printed or electronic form without permission. Please do not participate in or encourage piracy of copyrighted materials in violation of the authors' rights. Purchase only authorized editions.
Published simultaneously in Canada

Most Avery books are available at special quantity discounts for bulk purchase for sales promotions, premiums, fund-raising, and educational needs. Special books or book excerpts also can be created to fit specific needs. For details, write Penguin Group (USA) Inc. Special Markets, 375 Hudson Street, New York, NY 10014.

The Library of Congress has catalogued the hardcover edition as follows:

Ashton, Jennifer.
Your body beautiful : clockstopping secrets to staying healthy, strong, and sexy in your 30s, 40s, and beyond / Jennifer Ashton ; with Christine Rojo.
p.   cm.
Includes bibliographical references and index.
ISBN 978-1-58333-458-4
1. Women—Health and hygiene.   2. Physical fitness.   3. Health behavior.
I. Rojo, Christine.   II. Title.
RA778.A8325   2012   2011046402
613'.04244—dc23

ISBN 978-1-58333-510-9 (paperback edition)

Printed in the United States of America
10   9   8   7   6   5   4   3   2

BOOK DESIGN BY MEIGHAN CAVANAUGH

Neither the publisher nor the authors are engaged in rendering professional advice or services to the individual reader. The ideas, procedures, and suggestions contained in this book are not intended as a substitute for consulting with your physician. All matters regarding your health require medical supervision. Neither the authors nor the publisher shall be liable or responsible for any loss or damage allegedly arising from any information or suggestion in this book.

While the authors have made every effort to provide accurate telephone numbers, Internet addresses, and other contact information at the time of publication, neither the publisher nor the authors assume any responsibility for errors, or for changes that occur after publication. Further, the publisher does not have any control over and does not assume any responsibility for author or third-party websites or their content.

Dedicated to the memory of Dr. Reuben Zemel:

extraordinary surgeon, incredible teacher, kind friend, and

the first person who encouraged me to pursue my dream of

combining my love of medicine and my love of writing

CONTENTS

SECTION TWO

CLOCKSTOPPING SECRETS FOR LIFETIME WELLNESS

SECTION ONE

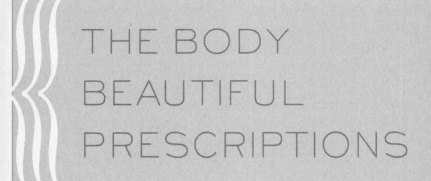

THE BODY BEAUTIFUL PRESCRIPTIONS

Five-Week Plans
to Transform Your Life

The Make-or-Break Years: Why Your Thirties and Forties Determine Your Lifetime Health

Not long ago, I spotted Jennifer Lopez at the grocery store. No, she wasn't in line with me at a New Jersey Stop & Shop, waiting to pay for her kids' Pull-Ups. She was on the cover of *People* magazine's "Most Beautiful People" issue.

I admit it: I couldn't wait to see who else made the list. As I flipped through, gazing enviously at the twelve gorgeous women in the issue, I noticed something shocking—and fabulous. Almost every single woman in those pages, with just a few exceptions, was in her thirties or forties (or even older!): J-Lo, forty-one; Sandra Bullock, forty-six; Dana Delany, fifty-five!

I was thrilled when I saw this—and it's not just because I'm forty-two! It's because the world has finally realized something that I've noticed for years in my medical practice as an ob-gyn. Many, many of my patients look (and *feel*) much better in their thirties and forties than they did in their twenties. The truth is, if you treat your body right, your thirties and forties can be your strongest, sexiest, most beautiful decades. Even better, the exact same habits that keep you healthy, strong, and sexy in your thirties and forties also lay the foundation for a lifetime of health and beauty, inside and out.

It's easy to overlook what a monumental realization this is. For as long as the modern media have been around, twenty-something women have gotten all the buzz. Everyone was supposed to look like they were under thirty. Even doctors weren't that interested in women after their late twenties, when they were theoretically done having babies (boy, *that's* changed!). After the last baby and before the first hot flash was a medical no-man's-land, when doctors put their patients on medical autopilot and didn't pay much attention to their health.

But today, *for the very first time in history,* the world in general, and doctors especially, are realizing that the thirties and forties are transformative decades for women. I don't just mean that these can be a woman's most beautiful years (although that's certainly true). Today, women in their thirties, forties, and beyond have more energy, vitality, and success than younger women. Consider this: When *Forbes* published a list of the world's fifty most powerful women in 2010, the vast majority, from Michelle Obama to Oprah, were in their forties or older.

It's no coincidence that the world is finally recognizing the incredible power of the thirties and forties in women's lives. In the past few years, new medical research has shown that these decades are the make-or-break years for health and beauty. If you're in your thirties or forties, you stand at a critical crossroads: You can put yourself on autopilot, because you're understandably preoccupied with work and family and too busy to pay much attention to your own health. Or, you can commit to building a specific set of habits, affecting how you eat, exercise, handle stress, and care for your skin, hair, and body. If you put in the work to develop these habits now, you can lay the foundation for a lifetime of health, strength, and physical and emotional beauty.

That's why I wrote this book. I want to take you step-by-step through a program to build the habits that will transform the rest of your life and keep your body beautiful, inside and out, for decades to come.

THE BODY BEAUTIFUL PHILOSOPHY

The thirties and forties are transformative decades. The habits you build now will lay the foundation for your health and beauty for the rest of your life.

The Magic of Habits

I'm the first to admit that the thirties and forties are a crazy period, between work, family, friends, pets, and everything else. Believe me, I know. I have two kids, two dogs, a husband with a demanding job, my own medical practice, and daily TV appearances as a medical correspondent. So I understand why my patients look at me like I'm nuts when I tell them they need to create a new set of eating, fitness, and stress-management habits. "Who has the time?" they ask me.

I answer: Who *doesn't*? You're too busy *not* to have healthy habits. The beauty of habits is that they're automatic. Once you've put in the work to develop them, they take care of themselves. They save time and effort because you don't have to think about them. Good health becomes a no-brainer. You automatically pick healthier foods. Your family takes it for granted that you're going out for a bike ride first thing in the morning. Your coworkers don't schedule you for lunchtime meetings on Tuesdays and Thursdays because they know that's when you hit the gym. These habits make you healthy, strong, and sexy in your thirties and forties *and* make you healthier for decades to come—you'll have more energy, more enthusiasm, be more productive, reduce sick time, and get more done. In other words, putting the time and effort in now to build healthy habits will save you time—and suffering—for the rest of your life.

That's why this book doesn't just tell you the latest research on good health and beauty. Instead, I give you specific steps designed to build good habits, five weeks at a time. None of these plans, not even my Five-Day/Two-Day diet, ask you to change overnight. Every single one of them has worked for me or my patients. They can work for you, too.

How to Use This Book

The newest research tells us that everyone builds habits at a different pace. One study asked ninety-six people to make a change in their eating, drinking, or exercising for twelve weeks, and monitored when that change became automatic—when it no longer took much effort to maintain. Results varied from eighteen days to nine months. The average was a little less than ten weeks.[1]

That's why this book is set up as a series of five-week programs, designed to be repeated until your new habits become second nature. Five weeks is enough time to start seeing and feeling real results. But five weeks *isn't* an impossibly long time—you can do *anything* for five weeks. By the time you repeat the five-week program another time (while also moving on to the next five-week plan, if you're ready), you'll have reached ten weeks, the average amount of time to build a habit.

The first section of the book is set up around the five areas where you need to develop healthy habits for life—the areas that have the biggest impact on your inner health and your outer beauty. These five areas are diet, fitness, beauty (especially sleep), stress reduction, and sex. You'll spend five weeks focusing on building new habits in each area, and then you'll maintain those habits as you move to the next area.

After about six months, you'll look and feel younger, stronger, and sexier—but, even more important, you'll have created new habits that will serve you for decades. Best of all, you'll know how to *create* new habits when you need them (because, over a lifetime, you'll need to change those habits as your body changes).

As you move through the chapters, you'll find more information giving you the latest research on why these habits work, along with additional approaches and tips that will help you look and feel your best. You'll also find clockstopping secrets, advice that's especially effective at stopping, slowing, or even reversing the clock on your appearance.

An important message is that every body is different, so every plan and set of habits will ultimately be different. The Body Beautiful program is about *finding* and *establishing* those habits that work best for you—not for your sister or for your best friend, but for *you*. After reading this, you may conclude that your eating or fitness habits are already right in line with all the newest research and working very well for you. Great. Move on to one of the other areas, like the five-week plan for better sex or stress management. In the future, you may find that one area or another has become a problem—you may be sleeping poorly, for instance—in which case you can return to the program just for that issue.

In the second section of the book, you'll find all the newest information on preventing disease, including cancer, heart disease, and more. These chapters will help you understand and evaluate your personal risks, and show you how the habits you're already working on with the five-week plans help protect you from the deadliest and most common diseases for women.

Building new habits in so many areas may seem daunting. But you'll quickly find that these habits all work together. When you're sleeping well, for instance, you're less stressed—and when you're practicing good stress-management habits, you'll sleep better. And all the five-week programs recommended here fit together in a holistic approach to total physical and emotional health designed to keep your body beautiful—for life.

The Body Beautiful Approach: Old-School Medicine with a New Age Approach

When I opened my own medical offices just for women a few years ago, I named the practice Hygeia, after the Greek goddess of health. I took enormous pride in designing an eco-friendly office, and a space that welcomes women as if they were coming to a spa, not to a cold, impersonal medical clinic. I don't make my patients wear paper robes that gape wide open—I give them comfy spa robes instead.

I tell my patients that my philosophy is "old-school medicine with a new age approach." When it comes to health and beauty, I believe we need to use every weapon in our arsenals to look and feel our best. That means paying attention to what we put in, and on, our bodies, and always choosing the purest, most natural approaches first. But when those don't work for our bodies, I believe in using the best, most recent, and most well-researched medical science and technology for the best results. So, throughout this book, you'll find information on natural, organic approaches to health and beauty, with a special emphasis on the Ayurvedic approach to wellness, which advocates simple, natural health care. You'll also find the very latest research and pro and con lists about health and beauty technologies, from cutting-edge cancer therapies to Botox. In the end, my job is not to judge your health choices, but to guide you in making smart, informed decisions based on what's right for you. After all, it's *your* body beautiful. Only *you* can make the choices that seem best for your own health.

Your Body in Its Thirties and Forties

The thirties and forties are a transformative time for many reasons. Sure, healthy habits were important in your twenties. But let's face it—you probably felt pretty good even without a lot of effort. Your body could bounce back easily from too many late nights, too much Ben & Jerry's, or that last tequila shot. It's like your body had training wheels back then. You could make lots of mistakes and keep cruising along. But by your thirties and forties the training wheels are off, and you need to learn real balance through sustainable health habits if you want a smooth ride through the coming years. That's what makes them such critical decades.

Unfortunately, most of us don't realize that we're riding with training wheels until they're gone and we fall down healthwise, eating junk food, putting on weight, letting stress eat away at us. That's why, in my office, not a week goes by without a patient coming in, shell-shocked, and saying, "My body is changing, and not for the better. I don't know what to do! I want my old body back!"

Sound familiar? Thirty years ago, your doctor would gently pat your hand and say, "That's what happens as you age, dear." Back then, most doctors looked at the mid-thirties and late forties as the years of medical cruise control. But now we know better. So I offer my patients this reassuring answer: "Actually, there's a *lot* you can do for your body right now. You may not get your old body back, but your *new* body can be *even better* than before."

What we know now that we didn't know then is that there are actually three distinct stages of health between thirty and fifty. Doctors used to think your health and wellness needs stayed steady throughout that whole long period. This couldn't be further from the reality of what we know today.

Your stage is a combination of your chronological age, your genetics, and your lifestyle and fertility choices, so see where you fit in.

STAGE 1: POTENTIALLY PREGNANT

If you're planning to have a baby (or another baby) sometime in the future, you're in stage 1, no matter what age you are. You'll need to know how to eat, exercise, and care for yourself in a way that protects your fertility and gives you the best shot at healthy weight gain during pregnancy and reasonable weight loss afterward. While information in every chapter applies to you, I'll focus on pregnancy advice in chapter 7.

Your Body in the Potentially Pregnant Stage

Hormones: You still have regular menstrual cycles and probably have no signs of hormonal imbalance, such as acne, excessive body hair, or darkened skin on the back of your neck or in your armpits. (If you do have these symptoms, talk to your doctor about them.)

Social: You're likely to have numerous friends who are in a similar life stage.

Mental: You're easily able to multitask, but may deal with PMS, depression, or anxiety. You may feel overwhelmed at times with work, family, or personal responsibilities.

Tips for the Potentially Pregnant Stage

• Even if a baby is not on your radar, treat your body as if it were. Remember that roughly 50 percent of all pregnancies in the United

States are unplanned. Women often take much better care of their bodies when they're pregnant or hoping to get pregnant. If you're thinking of having a baby, it pays to get yourself into optimal health as soon as possible. (Even if you're not thinking of it, you still deserve to be in top health!)

- Establish regular patterns of sleep and exercise.
- Get preventive health-care checkups regularly; get screened for STDs and diabetes yearly.
- Find a physician whom you like and trust.

STAGE 2: TRANSITION

You're in stage 2 if pregnancy is no longer on your radar, but you're not in the premenopause stage, where your menstrual patterns change or when you start having hot flashes or other symptoms. Women in transition often experience a burst of renewed energy that can last for years. But you need to learn to recognize subtle hormonal and metabolic changes and adopt new habits so you stay in charge of your body.

Your Body in the Transition Stage

Hormones/metabolism: Some women experience subtle hormonal and metabolic changes from their late thirties to mid-forties, but many do not. Although every woman is different and metabolic changes can start earlier or later, generally speaking, women in transition are still producing enough testosterone and estrogen to provide good payoff in muscle mass and stable weight. The hormonal changes that might be taking place include irregular periods, more PMS, a slight increase in body weight, or changes in hair thickness.

Social: Women in transition can be more stable than in earlier years. If they're mothers, their kids may be older or in school. Whether they have kids or not, their work and careers may be more established, with more regular, predictable hours. This can mean more time for exercise, regular sleep habits, and attention to wellness routines. This is also a time when women might expand the ages of their circle of friends and find that they can hang out with people in their late twenties or early thirties as easily as they can with people in their fifties or older.

Fitness: Because women in transition aren't experiencing the hormonal variations of pregnancy or premenopause, their metabolism is often stable. That means small efforts in exercise, nutrition, and sleep can have big rewards. Investment in one's body, health, and spirit now will yield significant benefits down the road.

Sex: This can run the gamut between long dry spells and the best sex ever. Many patients tell me they have no libido. Others express a renewed confidence and sexual security with knowing what they want and how to get it.

Tips for the Transition Stage

- Focus on good sleep habits (see chapter 4). Seventy million people in the United States have sleep problems, but *you* don't have to!
- Wear sunscreen every day. If you didn't start this habit years ago, start now!
- Assess your physical likes and dislikes about your body. You're not about to go through the physical turmoil of childbirth and you're not yet experiencing big hormonal changes, so this is a good time to take steps to preserve the good and improve the bad—now and for the rest of your life.

STAGE 3: PREMENOPAUSE

Some doctors consider you to be premenopausal as soon as you're done having your last baby, right up until your period stops. For many women, that's a decade or more. To me, it doesn't make sense to shuffle all women into one category—premenopausal—because your body in your mid-thirties is different from in your late forties. So my definition of this stage is flexible. If you're in your late forties and you are still having periods, you're in stage 3.

Your Body in the Premenopause Stage

Skin: During the premenopause stage, aging effects on your skin may become more pronounced. Skin becomes thinner and drier. The collagen in the under-layer (the subcutaneous layer) of skin becomes reduced and weaker, leading to less elasticity and more wrinkles. We'll talk about what you can do about that, and what you can't, in chapter 3.

Metabolism: Many women in the premenopause stage notice they've developed a "spare tire" of fat around their midsection. Your metabolism may slow down, causing you to gain weight even though your eating and exercise patterns have stayed stable. Many of my patients tell me they're sure they suddenly have an abnormal thyroid causing them to gain weight. While it's true that underactive thyroid gland activity is more commonly detected in women as they age (see chapter 8), the extra pounds may equally be caused by other types of hormonal changes. During premenopause, less estrogen circulates through the body, while testosterone levels tend to stay relatively stable (because most estrogen is made in the ovaries, but testosterone is made both in the ovaries and in the adrenal glands). At the same time, two androgens (precursors to "male" hormones), DHEA and DHEAS, drop to lower levels, which may contribute to changes in body fat. The body also produces less growth hormone as we age, which leads to less muscle mass and more body fat. Meanwhile, levels of a hormone called leptin—which sends you messages that you've eaten enough and you're full—decrease with age. It's not clear that this plays a role in weight gain, but it could certainly make you want to eat more than usual. These hormonal changes can also lead to other symptoms: disturbed sleep, erratic periods, even hot flashes. For more on hormonal changes and what you can do, see chapter 8.

Mental: As you approach menopause, you may feel more irritable, more tired/fatigued, more moody, and more anxious.

Sexual: All of the above changes may contribute to a decrease in libido or desire, as well as pain or problems with intercourse, including vaginal dryness and difficulty having an orgasm.

Tips for the Premenopause Stage

- Do *not* despair! You might be in the 10–15 percent of women who don't experience *any* menopausal symptoms. And even if you're not, those symptoms aren't here to stay. Most symptoms, like mood changes and altered bleeding patterns, are merely temporary, lasting an average of four years. I know that sounds like a long time, but in the chapters ahead, I'll tell you how to treat them.
- Don't fall for magic diet pills. It's still about the basics of physics: Calories *in* versus calories *out*. The equation may have changed, so it's crucial to figure out what works now. Maybe when you were younger, you could lose weight by altering just one side of the equation: eating less or exercising more. Now you have to do *both*: reduce the number of calories consumed, and increase the amount of energy burned by exercising more.

- Short-term changes don't work. Whether it's weight gain or other symptoms you want to control, shifting your metabolism is a long-term effort. But it's one that will pay off for the rest of your life.
- Control your metabolism now, before metabolic changes end up controlling you. In chapter 1, I'll explain fitness and nutrition strategies in detail. But for now, just remember that anticipating these metabolic changes *before* they occur can help you keep your body beautiful through midlife and beyond.

Forty Is the New Thirty

What I really want my patients, and you, to know is that forty really can be the new thirty, and fifty can be the new forty. The key to keeping your body beautiful is to do whatever it takes in your thirties and forties to develop a few lifetime habits that will lay the foundation for decades of inner and outer beauty. I'll give you lots of advice and encouragement and very specific steps to do that. But ultimately, it's up to you to take responsibility for your own future health. As I said earlier, it's *your* gorgeous, strong, healthy, sexy body, Beautiful. And only you can keep it that way.

1

The Five-Day/Two-Day Plan

For years, I thought my diet was pretty healthy. Okay, I'll admit, I never loved vegetables. And, true, when I was doing my medical training and after my kids were born, I was always on the run, grabbing a cookie here, a bagel there, or cramming down pizza without even noticing. It was only by accident that, six years ago, I suddenly discovered an eating plan that could keep me and my patients slimmer, healthier, and feeling great. I call it my Five-Day/Two-Day Plan.

The plan couldn't be simpler: Cultivate terrific eating habits (specifically, cut bad carbs and eat lots of veggies, fruits, and proteins) Monday through Friday, then take it easier on the weekends. Anybody can do it. By the end of five weeks, you'll have lost weight and, more important, started to establish long-term food habits that can keep you looking and feeling younger for the rest of your life.

You Can Do *Anything* for Five Days

It all started when my patient Jane needed to lose some weight before an elective surgery. I began researching diets for her, and I was astounded by how complicated, time-consuming, and expensive the most popular weight-loss programs seemed. Seriously—what woman in her thirties or forties has the time to log every single calorie or gram of carbohydrate or protein, or go to weekly meetings? Research shows these strategies can work for many people. But they do *not* fit the lives of women like Jane, a working mom in her late thirties with three kids and no extra time or money to spare. I wanted to find her a diet that was so simple, she could stick to it for the rest of her life.

A colleague told me he often puts his patients who need to lose weight quickly on a healthier version of a low-carb plan popular at the time: cutting out refined carbs (sugar, white bread, baked goods made with white flour) and starchy veggies (potatoes, corn, squash), but including lots of fruits, veggies, and lean proteins every day. It sounded good for Jane's short-term needs, but still too restrictive for the longer term. You can only deprive yourself for so long before falling off the wagon. But what if she did the diet during the week, then eased up and enjoyed her favorite foods in moderation on the weekends? Before recommending it to Jane, I tried it myself for a week.

On Monday, I announced to my husband, Rob, "I'm not eating bread, cereal, or bagels until Saturday." He assumed I was joking. He's a doctor and, like most doctors, highly skeptical of miracle diet plans. I immediately found myself on the receiving end of what would be a whole week of ridicule.

"You don't really think that's gonna work, do you?" he asked. "I mean, aren't you a doctor? How can you fall for some gimmicky diet? You'll never stick to it."

One week and three pounds later, he ate his words (pardon the pun). The next week, my husband was on the very same diet.

I share this story not because it's the best diet in the world, or because I love to point out the rare occasion when Rob is wrong. I tell this story because that experience transformed how Rob and I eat. We simply hadn't been paying much attention to what we put in our mouths, even though we knew better. Just one week of careful attention and effort led to major results. We looked better and felt better. Six years later, we still do.

After that week, we took stock of how we were eating. The plan had forced me into eating greens I'd always avoided, and it turned out I loved them. I also learned that if I avoided carbs in the form of bread, cereal, and pasta during the week, I lost weight.

Another thing we learned is that most diets fail in the long term because they're too structured and restrictive. As soon as you go off the diet, you gain the weight right back. But with the Five-Day/Two-Day Plan, you don't have to deprive yourself; you just have to be careful during the work week. When I first started the plan, I thought Saturday—and pizza night—would never come. But I told myself I could do anything for five days—and it turned out I really could! Then I stayed with it, saying I could stick to anything for five weeks. At the end of that time, my eating habits had changed permanently—and I'm still on the plan today.

Since then, the plan has worked for Jane and many, many other patients. It works well for several reasons. First, it's sustainable. Most people can do anything for five days. It's keeping something up forever that's hard. This plan works because those five days during the hectic week go by fast, and then you get to relax and eat a healthy, satisfying amount of the things you like best. It's also simple, which is important, because most of my patients in their thirties or forties don't have time for anything complicated.

Another reason it works is pure math. Over one year, you will spend 260 days being strict with your food choices, and only 104 days being more lenient—260 days wins! For the majority of the year, you'll be eating very healthfully.

The last reason it works is simple science. When you eat fewer carbs, your body's metabolism slowly changes. Initially, I found myself practically counting the minutes until the bagel store opened on Saturday mornings. That first bite after five breadless days was pure heaven. After a few months, though, I was surprised to notice that I had completely lost my cravings for bread, even on the looser two-day part of my week. So, sneakily and with no effort on my part, I found the five days of good behavior often accidentally became seven days. That's the nature of habits, after all: Once you make them, they're hard to break. Even the good habits!

CLOCKSTOPPING SECRET: SUGAR MAKES YOU LOOK OLDER

The Five-Day/Two-Day Plan calls for you to cut refined carbs, including sugar, out of your diet during the week. Not only does this help you avoid blood sugar spikes and lows, but it may help you look younger. A study published in the *British Journal of Dermatology* showed that sugar in the blood bonds with proteins to create harmful molecules that in turn damage other proteins, including collagen and elastin, which make your skin supple. The report showed that the aging effects of sugar become visible after age thirty-five and accelerate rapidly after that.[1] Turns out that sugar is anything but sweet to your face!

The Body Beautiful Prescription: Your Five-Day/Two-Day Plan

The Five-Day/Two-Day Plan helps you build healthy habits over five weeks. You'll make one very simple change in week one, then build on it by adding another good habit in week two, and so on. These aren't arbitrary, though: If you want to lose weight, you need to follow the changes in order and stick to them faithfully Monday through Friday. I know you can do it—it's only five days!

As with any diet, please check with your doctor about this plan and the supplements I recommend before diving in. See the section titled "Your Healthy Weight" to figure out a weight goal for yourself. It may take you a while to get there, but this plan will help make sure you stay there once you do!

WEEK 1: CUT BAD CARBS
MONDAY THROUGH FRIDAY

There's only one simple change you have to make this week. Eat as you normally would, but remove all bad carbs from your diet—that includes sugar (including high-fructose corn syrup), white flour, white rice, and pasta. That means no cookies, candy, crackers, cereal, bagels, bread, muffins, pretzels, chips, pizza crust, and so on. You can, however, eat carbohydrates in the form of fruits and vegetables—as much as you want! If you absolutely must have bread or pasta, choose whole-wheat varieties (and make sure the bread doesn't have sugar or corn syrup added), and if you must have rice, choose brown rice. However, for more effective results, pass them by completely until Saturday.

Why cut the carbs? Bad carbs are carbohydrates with the fiber removed. Your body absorbs these carbs more quickly, causing blood sugar spikes and making you hungrier faster. Good carbs (found in fruits, vegetables, and whole-grain products) contain fiber and take longer to digest. When you eliminate the bad carbs, you'll feel fuller and lose weight, while protecting your body from the negative impact of blood sugar spikes.

When the weekend comes, go back to eating what you enjoy in moderation (no bingeing!). Meanwhile, I want you to take three supplements every day: 1,000 IU of vitamin D_3, 1,000 mg of calcium (taken twice a day in doses of 500 mg each unless you get a lot of calcium from your diet), and 1,000 mg of omega-3 fatty acids. See the section titled "The Five-Day/Two-Day Supplements" for more information on supplements.

WEEK 2: DON'T DRINK YOUR CALORIES

This week, continue to avoid all the big offender carbs while making another change: Don't drink your calories. Just by cutting out sugar and bad carbs during week 1, you've already eliminated regular soda. But this week, I want you to cut out fruit juices, smoothies, alcohol, and lattes. Drink only zero-calorie beverages (water, seltzer, unsweetened tea, black coffee, etc.) until Saturday. Just one exception allowed: one cup of coffee with half-and-half a day. If you absolutely must drink soda or another sweet beverage, choose the zero-calorie or diet version. I don't like the chemicals in these drinks, but this week, the calories are more important. If the diet drinks help satisfy you, do it, but try to switch to healthier options without artificial sweeteners as soon as you can.

Cutting out liquid calories is a very simple change, but one that's made a huge difference for many of my patients. Last year, for instance, my patient Ashley came in for her first visit with me. She's a spunky five feet three inches, but she was rightly concerned about her weight. At forty-nine, she knew that her 231-pound bulk was contributing to borderline high blood pressure and putting her at increased risk for type 2 diabetes. I asked her my usual new-patient questions about diet and nutrition, and she mentioned that she drank five cups of coffee a day— big cups with half-and-half and lots of sugar.

I pulled out my calculator.

For Ashley, each creamy cup of joe was adding a whopping 200 calories to her diet. Multiply that times five, and that's 1,000 calories, just in coffee. That's like eating twenty Oreo cookies a day! Multiply by seven days—7,000 calories a week! Since 3,500 calories produce about a pound of fat, she could be losing two pounds a week if she cut out the cream and sugar!

I suggested she use 1 percent or skim milk and stevia sweetener in four of her five cups. One cup she should have exactly the way she liked it, half-and-half and all. I knew that if she deprived herself totally, she'd be less likely to sustain her new habit. According to my calculator, we figured this simple change could help her lose fifty-two pounds in just one year. That really got her attention.

Six months later, Ashley came back, thirteen pounds lighter simply from slightly changing her coffee pattern. She still has more changes she wants to make, but her story supports the rule I strongly emphasize to all my patients: *Don't drink your calories.* Wine, juice, cocktails—they all pack a big caloric punch. Plus, cutting back on the calories you drink is a change that's usually pretty easy to swallow—and the benefits are enormous.

LIQUID CALORIES

A rough approximation of the calories in your favorite
beverages . . . and what you could eat instead.[2]

2 percent milk, 8 oz.	120 calories, or one large apple
Orange juice, 8 oz.	110 calories, or 8 oz. of light, nonfat yogurt
Soda, 12 oz.	120–190 calories, or one slice of pepperoni pizza
Bottled iced tea, sweetened, 12 oz.	130–140 calories, or one small granola bar
Coffee with half-and-half (2 tablespoons)	40 calories, or one cup of whole strawberries
Low-fat latte, 8 oz.	120 calories, or two oat-bran mini-bagels
Beer, 12 oz.	150 calories, or ¾ cup light, no-sugar-added ice cream
Wine, 5 oz.	120 calories, or 2½ slices of low-fat cheddar cheese

WEEK 3: ADD A MID-MORNING
PROTEIN SNACK

Now you've dealt with the worst of the bad habits and you've probably
lost a few pounds (if you haven't, skip down to the section on portion
size). As you develop new positive habits, it's important to reward yourself. This is a time in the eating plan where you may start to falter, so
instead of cutting something out, you add in a treat: a mid-morning
protein snack to help you feel full and keep you going until lunch. For
your protein snack, choose either plain, low-fat Greek yogurt, a handful

of almonds, or a hard-boiled egg. This will help prevent blood sugar lows and let you avoid the cravings that lead to bingeing. Adding protein now will help you keep off the weight you've lost while helping to keep you full.

WEEK 4: ADD COLORS TO YOUR PLATE

Now that you've really picked up momentum and mastered the key habits to losing weight (cutting bad carbs, not drinking calories, and adding protein to stay full), this is the time to take it to a more advanced level. At every meal this week, make sure you have two or three colors on your plate. By *colors*, I really mean fruits and vegetables, the more, the better. In fact, you can eat unlimited amounts of your colors. That means as much broccoli, as many strawberries, as many carrots, as you want. This is the simplest way to guarantee that you're getting a variety of nutrients from a variety of sources.

Fruits and veggies are high in fiber and really fill you up, so you don't get as hungry later. Even more important, eating a wide variety of fruits and vegetables is one of the healthiest lifetime eating habits you can develop. Over the years, it will transform you outside as well as inside, giving you better health, helping prevent disease, and improving your energy, hair, skin, and weight.

WEEK 5: ADD AN AFTERNOON PROTEIN BOOSTER

At this point, you've stripped out all the bad habits and added some great ones. In this final week of the five-week plan, add another treat— a protein shake in the afternoon. I have one every day, and it keeps me going until dinner. Like a mid-morning snack, this will help you feel full and satisfied and avoid the feelings of deprivation that lead to cheating, bingeing, and other bad habits. (Note: This doesn't violate the "don't drink your calories" rule, because it's really a mini-meal, not empty carbs and calories.)

This is my favorite protein shake recipe, but you can develop your own.

Dr. Ashton's Protein Booster

Plant-based protein powder, amount as instructed on package (I use a brand called Vega, available at Whole Foods Market)

Water, amount as instructed on protein powder package

½ banana

4–6 large frozen strawberries (make sure they don't have sugar added!)

½ cup frozen spinach

Blend it all together and enjoy!

Note: Be sure to wait until week 5 to add the protein shake! If you haven't cut out the bad carbs and developed the other healthy habits first, you won't lose weight.

CHECK IN WITH YOUR BODY— AND KEEP GOING, FOR LIFE!

At the end of five weeks, you'll find changes that seemed difficult at first are now just habits. Take a moment to congratulate yourself and assess your progress. How do you feel and look? Have you lost weight, or maintained the weight you wanted? How did you do on the weekends?

You'll find that now you're automatically picking the right foods and making better choices. If you haven't reached your goal, try writing down everything you eat. (Yes, even if you slip and have a doughnut or a sundae, write it down. Do *not* waste your energy feeling guilty or beating yourself up! Just record it and move on.) Then look over your journal at the end of the week and see where you slipped up and why. Were you really hungry? Were you stressed? Think of substitutions: If you ate chips, try carrots instead. If you were eating because you were bored or tense, try a quick walk around the block to clear your head. You know yourself better than any weight-loss program ever could, so you're the best person to troubleshoot your eating patterns. If the past five weeks didn't result in any weight loss, don't despair! Keep up these habits; they *will* pay off! I promise.

The Five-Day/Two-Day Supplements: Vitamin D₃, Calcium, and Omega-3 Fatty Acids

Every year it seems there's some new miracle vitamin—and some new study debunking last year's pet nutrient. In the end, I recommend most of my patients take just three vitamins, which I mentioned earlier. Here's what they are and why you should take them. Be sure to talk to your doctor, though, before taking supplements (especially vitamin D_3—see my note below).

Vitamin D_3: Take 1,000 IU a day. Naturally available from fatty fish like salmon, herring, and sardines (my favorite), vitamin D_3 is the active form of Vitamin D, which is critical for bone health and function, and thought to be essential for good immune function. Higher levels of vitamin D in the blood have been associated with protection from cancer, heart disease, depression, and even diabetes. Vitamin D is also available from fortified milk, breads and cereals, and sun exposure—about fifteen minutes a day of direct sunlight—but unfortunately, sunscreen seems to reduce the body's ability to absorb vitamin D. Since sun exposure also causes skin damage and can lead to skin cancer, I feel it's safer to get your vitamin D from natural food sources or supplements.

Take a look at your calcium supplement, which may already include vitamin D_3, to make sure you don't overdose. Megadoses of vitamin D_3 (say, 10,000–50,000 IU a day) for many years can lead to high levels of calcium in the blood, as well as nausea, vomiting, and other unpleasant symptoms.

For people with a history of kidney stones, like myself, even lower doses of vitamin D_3 (2,000 IU a day or less) can increase the formation of kidney stones, so discuss vitamins with your doctor. On the other hand, certain medications, such as anticonvulsants, cholesterol-lowering medications, and certain antifungal treatments, can affect your body's vitamin D production. For people taking any of these medications, a supplement may be even more important.

Calcium: Take 1,000 mg a day, divided into morning and evening doses of 500 mg each. Recent studies have shown that women taking extra calcium in supplement form may be at higher risk of heart attacks, but calcium is important for strong bones. As with any other supplement, it's best to get your calcium directly from food sources like milk, sardines, and green leafy kale, but taking a supplement will make sure you get what you need. The body can't absorb too much calcium at one time, so dividing the dose into two is better than taking it all at once.

Omega-3 fatty acids: Take 1,000 mg a day. Omega-3 fatty acids containing EPA and DHA have been associated with heart and brain protection as we age. Too much can increase the risk of bleeding, so stick to the recommended amount. Keeping them in the refrigerator may reduce the chance that they will repeat on you (that is, that you'll be burping fish all day!).

YOUR HEALTHY WEIGHT

Every body is different, and everyone has her own healthy weight. To see if you're in a healthy zone, doctors look at the ratio of your height and weight, then compare it to other people like yourself to determine your body mass index (BMI). Typically, the lower your BMI, the less body fat you have. For adults over twenty, a BMI of 18.5 to 24.9 is considered healthy. That still leaves a very broad range. For a woman who's five feet five inches, a healthy BMI ranges from 111 to 150 pounds. To calculate your healthy BMI, go to the Centers for Disease Control website at www.cdc.gov and search *body mass index*. Note that while BMI is a reliable indicator of healthy weight for most people, it can be off-kilter for athletes (the BMI calculation may overestimate their body fat) and for older people who have lost muscle over the years (BMI calculators may underestimate their body fat).[3]

If you find you have a large amount of weight to lose, don't be discouraged. Losing even 5 percent of your body weight can start to yield big health dividends, so be proud of every pound! Even if it takes months before you see a difference, and a year to reach your goal, healthy changes are happening inside your body—and you'll enjoy the results for the rest of your life.

CLOCKSTOPPING SECRET: BEING TOO THIN MAKES YOU LOOK OLDER

If you're at the higher end of your healthy BMI, don't feel you have to lose more weight to look even better or younger. In fact, being too thin ages your face, according to researchers at Case Western Reserve University School of Medicine. In a recent study of two hundred identical twins, they found that twins over forty who'd lost too much weight looked older than their siblings. "Try to keep your weight around the ideal range, and if you do that, you'll look younger than if you lose a lot of weight," Dr. Bahman Guyuron, author of the study, told reporters.[4] One more reason to avoid fad diets and find sustainable lifetime habits that keep you looking and feeling your best—and youngest!

The Five-Day/Two-Day Plan: How It Works for Me

I've been on the plan for six years, and I've learned a lot about my body. For instance, I found I feel best when I eat every three hours. A typical day for me looks like this:

BREAKFAST:
- One slice of sprouted whole-grain bread with peanut butter (lots of protein!)
- Coffee with half-and-half
- A big glass of water

Mid-Morning Snack: Low-fat, plain Greek-style yogurt with a big glass of water

Lunch: Salad with grilled chicken, apples, and dried cranberries. A glass of seltzer water on ice.

Afternoon Snack: Homemade protein shake

All Day: Several glasses of water

Dinner: Grilled chicken or fish with broccoli, salad, or quinoa. Seltzer with lime.

TGIF! MY WEEKEND PLAN

At the start of the diet, when Saturday came, I was first in line at the bagel shop. I couldn't wait for that first bite—and, boy, was it wonderful. Over time, though, I found my eating habits had changed so much, I just didn't crave carbs like I used to. Now, on the weekends, I'll usually have a glass of wine on both nights, I might treat myself to a scoop of vanilla ice cream for dessert, and I'll happily eat sushi with white rice. I also don't guilt myself. If my daughter bakes a cake, I'll eat some—but I take a small portion. Because I eat small meals or snacks every three hours instead of having giant meals three times a day, I get full pretty fast, because my stomach's not stretched out and it's easier to stop after small portions.

Tips for Success

THE TWO-HAND RULE: DOWNSIZE YOUR PORTIONS

If you've been on the plan for three weeks and haven't lost weight, check your portion size. My rule of thumb is simple: No meal should be more than the amount of food you can cup between two hands. (Note: That's your *whole* meal—meat, side dish, everything *except* veggies. You can eat all the veggies you want.) Look at your hands. That doesn't look like it would be a whole lot of food, does it? That's because we have *lost our minds* in this country about what an appropriately sized serving of food really is. Visit any chain restaurant, order an entrée meant for one, and you'll get a meal that could easily feed a family of four.

This suddenly became glaringly clear on January 1, 2011, when chain restaurants were required to start putting their calorie counts on the menus. A chicken burrito with all the fixings and a side of chips at Chipotle—1,780 calories! That's almost a full day of calories based on the USDA's recommended average daily calorie intake of 2,000 calories! A large tuna melt at Quiznos—1,520 calories. A Santa Fe Chicken Salad from Applebee's—a *salad,* mind you!—is 1,310 calories.

Is it any wonder that 60 percent of adults in the United States are overweight or obese?

Don't fall into this supersized trap. It's easy to avoid if you remember the two-hand rule. You might still feel hungry when you finish, but you'll feel full soon—it takes a while for our brains to catch up with our stomachs when it comes to feeling full.

Other simple ways to monitor your portion size:

- Use smaller plates when eating at home. A smaller plate holds less food, but makes it look like more than a larger one would.
- Eat the lower-calorie foods on your plate first before starting on the more calorie-rich items. You won't be as hungry when you get to the fattening stuff.
- When serving yourself at home, if you'd normally dish out two scoops of something, take only one.

SHOPPING CART MAKEOVER

Willpower is *not* my strong point. If there's a cookie anywhere in my house, I'll eat it. If not, I don't even think about it. So sticking to my

Five-Day/Two-Day Plan is infinitely easier if I make sure the high-calorie foods never see my kitchen. That means keeping them out of the shopping cart. If you fill up your cart with vegetables and fruits, you'll fill your tummy with them as well. Stick to a list of healthy basics that fit into your plan (I've started your shopping list for you below). Then, when you shop, hug the edges of the supermarket—the produce bins, the meat and fish sections, the milk and eggs shelf—and avoid the middle aisles, where they stock all the "factory food," like chips, cookies, and other prepackaged selections. Better yet, go to a farmers' market. Not a single bag of chips in sight!

YOUR FIVE-DAY/TWO-DAY SHOPPING LIST

- Fresh fruits and vegetables (if it's winter, try frozen fruits and veggies, but make sure they don't have added sugar)
- Fresh herbs (basil, cilantro, rosemary, and dill make a big difference on grilled fish or meat)
- Nonfat yogurt and milk
- Low-fat cheese
- Eggs or egg substitute
- Whole-wheat breads with no high-fructose corn syrup added
- Whole-wheat tortillas (great for wraps with turkey and lettuce)
- Low-fat broth
- Vegetable soups (avoid cream-based soups)
- Balsamic vinegar (makes a great no-calorie dressing)
- Hummus (terrific with fresh vegetables—great substitute for chips and salsa)
- Seltzer water (satisfying and filling, especially with a splash of lime or lemon)

AVOID PACKAGED FOODS

If you've mastered the five-week plan, and you're now maintaining your good habits, here's an added challenge that can really transform your eating: Try to go an entire week without eating packaged foods. No boxes of cereal or crackers, not even a bag of vegetables. Spending just one week avoiding packages altogether will make you more aware of how much of our diet comes from factories, not farms—and, almost by definition, by avoiding packaged foods, you'll avoid extra fat, sugar, carbs, and preservatives.

RULES FOR RESTAURANTS

I love to eat out, but it didn't take me long to realize that one restaurant meal, even a seemingly healthy one, could knock me off my eating plan. The same is true for travel. When I'm on the road, it's really tempting just to eat whatever's convenient. Next time you're traveling or have a week when you're eating out a lot, follow these rules:

- Ask the server not to bring bread.
- Order an appetizer as your main course, or split your entrée with a friend.
- Order two appetizers instead of an appetizer and a main course.
- Ask for substitutions. Can you get fruit instead of hash browns? Carrots instead of fries?
- Order soup (as long as it's not creamy). Soup is filling and usually relatively low in calories compared to other menu items. Always ask the server if the soup has a cream base—if so, choose something else.
- Don't trust the salad! At some chain restaurants, the salads have more calories than the entrées! This is especially true of taco salads or any salad with a heavy dressing or lots of cheese or meat. If you

order salad, be sure it's mostly vegetables, and ask for a low-fat dressing on the side.

- Don't read the dessert menu. Ask for fresh fruit if you need a sweet treat at the end.

STEER CLEAR OF THE FEEDING TROUGH

Ironically, there's no greater threat to a doctor's health than the nurse's station. Any good doctor will tell you that nurses are the wind beneath our wings; they can make or break good medical care, and behind every good doctor is a great nurse. They help us take care of our patients, and often they even take care of us. They support us emotionally and they feed us—and lots of people feed them, too. Stop by any nurse's station and you'll find a cornucopia of mouthwatering treats, many high in fat, carbs, and sugar, ready to sustain health-care workers through grueling hours. Sound familiar? Many workplaces have a feeding trough some-where, especially around the holidays. Try to steer clear of these danger zones altogether, especially if you're hungry, tired, or stressed. Try bringing in healthier substitutes and making a pact with your coworkers to ban doughnuts and other high-fat treats.

ENJOY!

If you struggle with your weight (and who doesn't?), you probably hear two voices talking in your ears. One is telling you to eat less, to diet more, that food is bad. The other part wants to enjoy the primal pleasure of eating. Good news: One of the most important things you can do to stay healthy is to have a good relationship with your food, and that means really enjoying the act of eating. Food, after all, is one of life's great plea-sures, and one way to stick to good eating habits is to make sure you enjoy every minute of your eating experience.

In this domain, we can learn a lot from other parts of the world. In

India, for example, followers of Ayurvedic wellness traditions believe that eating should be a ritual of sorts. It should be relaxing, pleasant, and nutritious, without being rushed or stressed. The thinking is that food feeds the mind and spirit as well as the body, and should therefore appeal to all the senses and serve each individual's unique nutritional needs, determined by her age, body type, season of the year, and any specific conditions. It's a lovely way to think about food and what it means to our lives.

But you don't have to master an Eastern philosophy to learn to enjoy eating more. Here are a few simple rules to help you savor your supper (and all your other meals, too!):

- Eat only when you're hungry.
- Drink a large glass of water or seltzer before you eat so your brain doesn't confuse thirst for hunger signals. The brain's just not that smart when food is on the line.
- Eat slowly. This is one rule that most doctors ignore—probably because if we don't eat quickly at work, we may not eat at all! But that's no excuse. People who eat more slowly tend to eat less on average than people who bolt their food. It may be that the longer food is in contact with the taste buds, the more the brain's satiety and satisfaction center is activated. Try putting your fork or spoon down between each mouthful and actually enjoy what you're eating. Savor the tastes and flavors and enjoy the people with whom you are eating. Bon appétit!

Are You Addicted to Food?

New research has shown that people can be addicted to food through the same biological and physiological processes that cause drug, alcohol, and tobacco addiction. This may explain why it's not always so simple to "just say no" to the Oreos or ice cream sundae. For food addicts, it's not just a shortage of willpower.

It turns out that there are many ingredients in food that act to stimulate the addiction centers in our brains. Foods high in sugar or fat (and many foods contain both!) trigger the release of chemical neurotransmitters. MRIs of the brains of people who eat high-fat or high-sugar foods show activation in the same areas of the brain affected by drugs like heroin or opium. We call these areas the reward centers of the brain.[5] In addition, brains of obese individuals share some cellular similarities with those of drug addicts, which may make them crave certain foods that produce the above-mentioned effects, giving them a food "high."

People who are addicted to food often know that certain foods are particularly unhealthy, but eat them anyway. They may eat compulsively as a response to stress and anxiety instead of to hunger. They may always be on a diet, always cranky and frustrated at their inability to lose weight or eat well. They may have low self-esteem. Food addicts are often obsessed with activities having to do with food or dieting, and spend a lot of time focusing on these things.

Scientists at Yale University's Rudd Center for Food Policy and Obesity have devised a food addiction scale to assess whether or not someone falls into this category (similar to the tests we use to identify depression, drug addiction, or alcoholism).[6] These are the kinds of questions it includes:

- When I eat certain foods, I wind up eating more than I wanted.
- Avoiding or cutting down on certain foods bothers me.
- When I overeat, I feel sluggish or have no energy—and this happens a lot.
- At times, I have eaten certain foods or foods in such quantities

that the time I spent dealing with the resulting negative emotions kept me from other important tasks, like work or social events that I enjoy.

- Even though I was having emotional or physical issues, I kept consuming the same types of food or food in the same amount.
- I need to eat more and more to feel full or fulfilled or emotionally satisfied.
- When I cut down or stop eating certain foods, I have withdrawal symptoms such as anxiety or agitation. (A caffeine headache doesn't count.)
- My behavior concerning food and eating causes me enormous upset.
- Because of my issues with food and eating, I have significant problems in my life (work, health, family, or social life).

If you answered *yes* or *true* to four or more of these questions, or if you answered *yes* to the last two questions, you may have an addiction to food. Talk to your doctor and visit the Rudd Center website at www .yaleruddcenter.org for more complete information on food addiction.

The scientific support for food addiction, however, does not take the personal responsibility away from you: You're the one who will have to find support and manage your addiction if you want a healthy life. But the research does add to our understanding of obesity as a complex issue driven by behavioral, social, emotional, chemical, genetic, and environmental forces. Yes, obesity is related to what we eat, but also to *why* we eat, *how much* we eat, the ingredients in our food, and how our brains react to eating. More research about food addiction is under way. If you think you have a food addiction, talk to your doctor, and look into the twelve-step food-addiction programs available nationwide that offer help.

Going Green:
Vegetarian Eating

My patient Dora, forty-one, suffered from irritable bowel syndrome. She wanted to turn over a new leaf in terms of her diet and fitness level. She launched a new exercise regime and decided to become a vegetarian.

Today, about 3 percent of American adults call themselves vegetarian, and another 10 percent (or 33 million people) claim they follow a vegetarian-inclined diet.[7] Some people, like Dora, decide to eat a primarily plant-based diet for health reasons, and others choose this path for economic, religious, or ethical reasons. Whatever the motivation, this type of diet requires careful planning to make sure you're getting the nutrients you need, so you should talk to your doctor about your vegetarian diet.

The American Dietetic Association suggests following a vegetarian food pyramid, including two servings a day of fats and fruits; four servings a day of vegetables; five servings a day of nuts, legumes, and other high-protein foods; and six servings a day of grains.[8] As healthy as a vegetarian diet can be, it's easy for vegetarians to have nutritional deficits. Vegetarians need to be sure they're getting the right amounts of the following nutrients (of course, so do meat-eaters).

VITAMINS FOR VEGETARIANS

Vegetarians should take the same daily supplements I recommend for all my patients: 1,000 IU of vitamin D_3, 1,000 mg of calcium, and 1,000 mg of omega-3 fatty acids. In addition, they need vitamin B_{12}, iron, and protein, as I describe below.

Vitamin D: Vegetarian sources of vitamin D include soy and rice milk.

Calcium: Vegetarians who don't consume dairy products can find calcium in kale, broccoli, turnips, soy, and tofu.

Omega-3 fatty acids: Vegetarians who do not consume fish or eggs may have trouble getting enough of this in their diets, so supplements are especially important.

Vitamin B_{12}: Vegetarians should take 2.4 mg a day. Vitamin B_{12} is key for red blood cell production, but it's found almost entirely in animal products, so it can be especially difficult for vegetarians and vegans to consume. Sources include vitamin-enriched cereals and fortified soy products. I also tell my vegetarian patients to get some B_{12} by eating one of the following daily:

- ⅕ ounce (3 halves) English walnuts (these are the walnuts you'll usually find in grocery stores—they're not black walnuts)
- ¼ teaspoon flaxseed oil
- 1 teaspoon canola oil
- 1 teaspoon ground flaxseed

Iron: Vegetarians need twice as much iron in their diets as non-vegetarians, because iron is not easily absorbed from plant sources. Iron is found in beans, lentils, dark green leafy veggies, and some dried fruits. To better absorb the iron, it helps to eat iron-rich foods along with those that are high in vitamin C, like citrus fruits, tomatoes, and broccoli. Periodically having your doctor check your blood count and iron levels can help make sure you are getting enough from your diet.

Protein: Important for healthy muscles, skin, bones, and major bodily functions. Protein sources include soy products, nuts, whole grains, legumes, and plant-based meat substitutes. To figure out how much protein your body needs, divide your weight by 2.2, then multiply by 1 to 1.5. So, if you weigh 120 pounds, you need about 54–82 grams of protein a day. You can get this from foods that are high in the amino acid lysine. Eat two to three servings a day from the following list:

- ¼ cup peanuts
- ½ cup cooked beans—garbanzo, kidney, pinto, or navy
- ½ cup lentils
- ½ cup peas—split or green
- soy foods—1 cup edamame, tofu, tempeh, or soy milk, or 3 ounces soy meats
- 1 cup cooked quinoa

? DID YOU KNOW?
It's easy to spot a fad diet.

From time to time as you age, you may find you need to boost your weight-maintenance motivation by trying a new and different diet for a while. If so, watch out for fad diets that may be unsafe or scams. Simply put, stay away from any diet that includes less than 1,200 calories a day for women and 1,600 a day for men, anything where you are expected to lose more than 1.5–2 pounds a week, and anything that seems like you can't sustain it over the long term in normal life. If you can't sustain it, you'll put the pounds right back on.

Loving Your Body Beautiful

The Five-Day/Two-Day Plan is not guaranteed to turn you into a supermodel. It's designed to help you reach and maintain the ideal, healthy weight for your body (which is not the ideal weight for waifs in a fashion magazine). Lots of my patients are at a healthy weight and exercise regularly, but still have their own complaints about their shapes. I tell them the important thing is that they're truly healthy, inside and out.

Here's what I *can* promise you: Even if you don't lose a single pound on this plan (which would be surprising!), your body will be much healthier for it. And as a doctor, that's what I care about most: I want you to be beautiful on the *inside*. Those inner changes aren't as inspiring or exciting because you can't see them and might not even feel them right away. But the eating habits I've outlined here will transform your inner self, helping to prevent disease and making your whole body work the way it should for years to come. Building these habits now, while you're still in your thirties and forties, can lay the foundation for decades of good health later. It's your body, Beautiful. Only you can choose the foods and eating habits that will keep it that way.

2

Sleek, Strong, Sexy

The Five-Week Workout Prescription

n my mid-thirties, I thought I was pretty fit. I'd always liked exercise, and even after having my kids, I managed to lift weights a few days a week. I didn't do much (okay, *any*) cardio because I had had knee surgery in my twenties. Frankly, as a mom with two jobs (as a doctor and a medical correspondent), I was proud of myself for working out *at all*. I thought if I could just keep squeezing in my weight-lifting sessions, I'd be set for life. No problem, I thought.

Then I met Dara Torres.

This amazing, gorgeous Olympic swimmer is still breaking records in her forties. She's sleek, strong, and sexy, and she looks ten times better than most women twenty years her junior. And those abs! To me, she was the living proof of everything I knew, intellectually, about exercise: It really *can* keep you strong, sexy, healthy, and gorgeous far into midlife and beyond. I came away from my talk with Dara completely inspired. I'd been on a fitness plateau, and now I was ready for a new approach to exercise.

Fortunately, at the same moment I was looking for a way out of my rut, I came upon a wave of research showing new ways to get more out of your workout time—essential for busy women.

Specifically, three new principles informed the plan I eventually came up with to get me out of my rut—a plan that helped me finish my first triathlon, at age forty-two, and introduced me to great new activities, including karate and the Bar Method. If you follow the plan, I promise you'll get more benefit in less time than you think and, even more important, have a lot more fun being active—and that's the key to creating active habits for a lifetime.

The three principles of the plan are:

1. **Work out smarter, not harder or longer.** Lots of research now shows that the body quickly adjusts to any routine, no matter how hard or long it is. But if you change your workout, constantly varying your pace, doing different activities on different days, or even working out on different surfaces (grass, pavement, trampoline, etc.), your body doesn't have a chance to get used to one routine, so you burn more calories in the same or even less time. This is great news for women in their thirties and forties. We're so busy with careers and/or family . . . who has time to work out more? If you add variety through interval training, which I'll explain, you'll get a better burn in less time.

2. **Make your muscles burn more calories when you're watching TV.** Muscle burns more calories than fat. So when you replace fat with muscle through weight training, you burn more calories even when you're just sitting around. This is why I tell my patients that weight training is the best-kept secret of women's health. When you work out with weights three times a week, your body burns more calories *all the time*. That's a great payoff for a couple of hours a week.

3. **Change is good . . . very good.** Lots of my patients have been running since college and think that's all they'll ever need. Actually, we now know our bodies need many different types of exercise, or they easily adjust to what we're doing and we lose the benefit. And we lose our motivation to improve.

These three principles sound simple, and they are. But they can transform your fitness routine and your body. The key is to establish new habits. But in this case, one of those new habits is going to be learning to *break* habits—always adding, exploring, and changing your routine so you never get bored, always stay motivated, and never fall into a fitness rut. Your end goal is to be alternating days of cardio intervals with days of weight training, plus a couple of wild card days where you add a new activity strictly for fun. The plan below will help you plan your workout.

CLOCKSTOPPING SECRET: EXERCISE MAKES YOUR CELLS YOUNGER

Studies show that people who work out regularly look younger—under the microscope, that is.[1] One study of twins found that people who worked out moderately to vigorously several times a week had cells resembling those of people ten years younger who didn't exercise.[2] The specific difference was in the length of something called *telomeres*, which are found at the ends of chromosomes. They work like the little plastic things at the ends of your shoelaces, keeping the laces from unraveling. When cells divide, telomeres get shorter; when they're too short, the cells can no longer divide, and they die. So just a few hours of exercise a week can keep your cells (and you!) looking younger!

STEALING TIME

One of my patients, who works as a receptionist in a dentist's office, was struggling to find time to exercise. Then she came up with a great plan: Once every sixty minutes at work, she takes a five-minute break, goes into the lunch room, and does ten squats, ten push-ups, and ten calf raises. By the end of the day, she's gotten in a half-hour weight routine. Her boss approved and her coworkers were inspired by her creativity.

Keeping Up with Changes:
Your Body at Thirty, Forty, and Fifty

Lots of my patients think they can keep following the same workout routine for their entire lives. They ran, swam, or biked in college, and they intend to do exactly the same for the rest of their lives. But thanks to the way your body changes, you need to make over your workout periodically, building new habits to fit your changing body.

In your thirties: If you had good eating and exercise habits in your twenties, your thirties will probably be fairly stable (with the possible exception of a few pregnancies). But if you partied your way through your twenties, you probably had a rude awakening at the big three-oh. Suddenly, you had to log in more hours at the gym to maintain the same body weight. Blame your slowing metabolism: a 1–2 percent decrease in the basal metabolic rate (BMR) each decade starting at age twenty. If you already had a good base of eating and exercising habits, though, small adjustments can make this change barely noticeable.

In your forties: Subtle hormonal changes and gravity start to change the shape of your body. Even if you weigh the same, you may look heavier. Your percentage of body fat increases, your percentage of lean muscle mass decreases, and inches sneak on where you don't want them. With muscle turning to fat, and fat heading south thanks to gravity, you can start to look rounder even if the number on the scale doesn't budge. Add weight training to your routine two or three times a week to help your body adjust to your changing metabolism and stave off osteoporosis.

By fifty: This is not the time to slow down. In fact, you need to exercise more (and eat less) to keep off the pounds. According to a study done at the University of Pittsburgh, most women gain an average of twelve pounds during the eight years after menopause. If in the past you lost or maintained weight by either eating less or exercising more, now you'll find it takes both just to maintain your weight. But don't get discouraged by this change. Remember the benefits of staying fit for your whole life—a more beautiful body, lower risk for many diseases, and a higher possibility of a longer, more energetic life—and pump it up!

The Concepts Behind the Five-Week Workout

Before I give you the actual week-by-week plan, you need to understand the magic of two exercise concepts: high intensity interval training (HIT for short) and weight training. When you see how these work, you'll understand how you can get more benefit from less time by following this plan.

HIT: THE PERFECT BUSY WOMAN'S WORKOUT

The cardio portion of the Body Beautiful plan is based on doing high intensity intervals. That's because new research shows that high intensity intervals can help you become much more fit in *less* time. Here's why: The trick with cardio is that your body gets very smart, very fast. It also gets bored quickly. As soon as your exercise routine feels comfortable and easy, it's a safe bet you've hit a plateau. You'd probably love to stay there. After all, it's flat. It has a lovely view. But it's not what you need, especially as you age. If your body's bored and not challenged by its exercise routine, you're not stressing your muscles. So what you need to do is add stress, not time, through interval training.

Interval training is brief, intense bursts of aerobic exercise (fast walking, running, biking, swimming, or using the elliptical). In a typical HIT workout, you might walk briskly for four minutes, then run for a minute, then repeat. Or you might jog for four minutes, then sprint for one. The important thing when you do HIT is that you really have to feel the burn. During the intervals when you are pushing yourself, really go for it. Work as hard as you possibly can for that one or two minutes.

When people exercise using these short but intense bursts or sprints, they reap all kinds of benefits, from burning more fat to rapidly increasing their endurance.[3] What's more, workouts can be short while still giving greater benefits than longer routines. Imagine: Doing twenty minutes of jog-sprint intervals four times a week can do more for you than jogging four days a week for an hour each time. You've just saved yourself lots of time *and* increased your fitness!

You're also doing lots to protect your body in the future. Studies have shown that interval training benefits muscles and improves both the structure and function of your blood vessels.[4] As you age, the flexibility of your blood vessels, both your arteries and your veins, decreases. This can affect your blood pressure, your circulation, and your heart, forcing it to work harder to pump against stiffer arteries. Intervals help prevent much of this trauma.

If interval training sounds like a lot of work—well, it is! But remember, you're actually going to reap greater benefits in *less* time. It's the perfect busy woman's workout.

CLOCKSTOPPING SECRET: EXERCISE BOOSTS MUSCLE STEM CELLS, KEEPING MUSCLES YOUNGER

Studies show that endurance exercise like running, swimming, and biking boosts the number of muscle stem cells that help rejuvenate muscles and protect against the loss of muscle mass and function that come with age. In one study, younger and older rats ran on a treadmill for twenty minutes a day for thirteen weeks; the younger rats showed a 20–35 percent increase in stem cells per muscle fiber, and older rats did even better, with a 33–47 percent increase.[5] This may explain why people who exercise regularly look and feel younger than those who don't: Their muscles really are younger.

THE STRENGTHS OF STRENGTH TRAINING: BURN MORE CALORIES ALL DAY LONG

Strength training is far and away the best-kept secret to keeping your body beautiful. Many of my patients have never tried it because they find the gym intimidating, worry about bulking up, or feel they'd burn more calories with cardio.

The truth is, weight training doesn't take very long, is a terrific activity for women, gives you gorgeous, sleek muscles (I've never seen a woman bulk up like a weight lifter unless she wanted to), and can actu-ally make your cardio workout much more effective. You're also getting a two-for-one fitness boost. First, as you slowly and subtly increase your muscle mass through strength training, you burn more calories even when you're resting. That's because muscle burns more calories than fat, even when you're watching TV. It turns up your basal metabolic rate.

Second, any weight-bearing exercise helps build bone density. Pump-ing iron stresses our bones—in a positive way—which stimulates them to develop more density, which combats osteoporosis. At the end of this chapter, I give you specific weight-training routines to follow, but most gyms will be happy to provide you with a trainer for your first visit or two to show you the ropes.

SECRET FOR EXERCISE BEGINNERS: YOU'LL BENEFIT MORE, FASTER, THAN YOUR FITTER SISTER

Many of my patients who are overweight are almost afraid to start exer-cising. They find it embarrassing. I say they should be proud instead. And if it's any help, I say, they'll reap bigger benefits faster than long-time exercisers! People who are moderately overweight enjoy huge ben-efits for losing just 5–10 percent of their starting weight. Say a woman who's five feet two inches and 160 pounds loses just 8 to 16 pounds. Her risk of chronic diseases, including high blood pressure and diabetes, goes down by 20–75 percent.[6]

To start an exercise routine, I recommend half an hour of walking every day. Plus, if you're not comfortable showing up at the gym, try a video like *The Bar Method* or any of a wide variety of yoga DVDs. After just a few weeks of daily walking and doing a tape, you'll be ready to try my five-week workout.

HOW MUCH IS ENOUGH?

The American Heart Association recommends a minimum of either two and a half hours a week of moderate exercise (where you breathe harder) or seventy-five minutes a week of strenuous exercise (where you really sweat). If you do the routine I recommend, you'll be achieving that goal. But there are other ways, too—daily walking, swimming, or moving in any way at all is better than nothing.

Remember these three rules: Repeat them out loud anytime you feel like you don't have time or motivation to exercise:

1. Some exercise is better than no exercise.
2. More exercise is better than less exercise.
3. Every minute counts.

If you can only get out jogging for ten minutes, do it. Standing is better than sitting, jogging is better than walking, walking is better than riding (in an elevator or on an escalator). What matters is that you do something as often as possible. If you can't do an official workout, you might walk up and down the stairs at work, or do push-ups or sit-ups while watching TV. Walk the dog and jog on the way home. Just get moving.

The Body Beautiful Prescription: Your Five-Week Workout

Like my other Body Beautiful prescriptions, the Body Beautiful workout is based on five-week segments to help you build new habits. But since variety is the spice of life—*and* the secret to a strong, sleek, sexy body—you'll change your main activity every five weeks.

A couple of notes:

- For convenience, I've referred to specific days of the week below. Obviously, you should pick the days that work for you.
- I've put my description of specific weight-training exercises at the end of the chapter.

WEEK 1: WARMING UP

Step 1: Commit to Three or Four Workouts This Week

Look at your calendar and write down your plan. Lots of research shows that writing down goals makes you more likely to achieve them. Most of my patients tell me the only way to make this work is to exercise first thing in the morning, before they start making excuses. Try getting up just forty-five minutes earlier (it's only for five weeks—you can do *anything* for five weeks!). I've written this week's plan for four days, but if you can only do three, start there, with two cardios and one weight session, and add another next week.

Step 2: Monday and Wednesday: Cardio Interval Training

Pick your favorite cardio workout. It could be walking, running, swimming, biking, the elliptical trainer, or spinning. You'll stay with this cardio routine for five weeks, then move on to another one.

For beginners: 1 minute walking, 1 minute jogging or brisker walking. Start with walking, either on a treadmill or outdoors. Walk for one minute at a normal pace, then jog or walk as fast as you can for one minute. Keep up this one minute on, one minute off routine for 20–25 minutes.

For moderate/advanced exercisers: 5 minutes jogging, 1 minute sprinting. Start out at your usual, moderate pace for 5 minutes, then add a 1-minute sprint. (If you're on a treadmill, stationary bike, or elliptical trainer, you can choose to change the resistance or incline rather than going faster.) Recover by returning to your normal pace (or lowering the incline or resistance) for another five minutes. Do this for 20 to 25 minutes.

Swimmers: If you're a lap swimmer, vary your routine by alternating strokes; say, 4 laps of freestyle, followed by 1 lap of butterfly, followed by 4 laps of breaststroke. Or, swim 4 laps at a fast pace, and then rest 20 seconds. Repeat this five times. For specific routines, look up swimming workouts on the U.S. Masters Swimming website at www.usms.org.

Experienced exercisers often worry about varying slow and fast segments instead of keeping a constant pace, fearing they'll benefit less because they slow down during recovery time. Don't worry—even with your recovery time, your heart is reaping the benefits.

Step 3: Tuesday and Thursday: Weight Training

Start with a 15–20 minute cardio warm-up of medium intensity. Beginners can walk on the treadmill; more experienced exercisers might try the elliptical or bike. The point here isn't to push yourself hard (you did that yesterday and you'll do it tomorrow); it's to get your muscles warm and loose.

Beginners: Do all six of the exercises described in the weight-training section. Start with 8 repetitions, then move on to the next exercise.

When you've done them all, go back to the beginning and do another set of 8.

Advanced: Do all six of the exercises described in the weight-training section. Do 12–15 repetitions of each, then start the cycle again, then one more time, so you've done three sets. If you find these are too easy and you're not tired after 15 reps, add more weight.

WEEK 2: BUILDING STRENGTH

Step 1: Add an Extra Workout Day to Your Calendar

If you did three last week, make it four this week. If you did four, make this week five. Again, write down what you intend to do on the calendar (then check it off when you're done—it feels great!).

Step 2: Monday, Wednesday, Friday: Cardio Interval Training

Beginners: 2 minutes slow, 1.5 minutes fast. This week, make your slower periods 2 minutes, with 1.5 minutes of fast walking or jogging. Repeat for 20–25 minutes.

Advanced: 4 minutes moderate, 1 minute sprinting. Reduce the amount of time between your sprints by 1 minute, so you're now jogging (or biking or swimming) at a moderate pace for 4 minutes, followed by your 1-minute sprint.

Step 3: Tuesday and Thursday: Weight Training

Beginners: Repeat the weight routine from week 1, but increase your reps; your goal is to reach 12–15 reps, doing two to three sets each.

Advanced: Repeat the weight routine from week 1, adding weight until it's difficult to do 12–15 reps, for three sets.

WEEKS 3–4: ADD CHALLENGES

Step 1: Add More Workout Days

Mark five days of exercise on your calendar this week, plus a wild card day when you try a new activity.

Step 2: Monday, Wednesday, Friday: Cardio Interval Training

Beginners: Increase your workout to 30 minutes. Make your sprints 2 minutes and your recovery period 2–3 minutes. If you've been walking briskly for your sprint intervals, try jogging if it's comfortable.

Advanced: Increase your workout to 30 minutes or more. Increase your sprint time and/or decrease your recovery time by 30 seconds.

Step 3: Tuesday and Thursday: Weight Training

Work with the weight levels from last week, adding reps or sets as you can. Add the balance challenges listed below to engage more muscles and get a better workout in the same amount of time.

Step 4: Wild Card Day: New Workout

In weeks 3 and 4, add a sixth day of activity—this can be anything, as long as it's new. Rock climbing, karate, yoga, ballroom dancing, Zumba class, an exercise video—anything you've been curious to try. If you used to play soccer, get out a ball and kick it around with friends and family. The idea here is to test out different kinds of activities.

WEEK 5: THE GRAND FINALE

Step 1: Monday, Wednesday, Friday: Cardio Interval Training

Really push it this week. Try 3-minute sprints and 2 minutes of recovery for 30 minutes total. Remember, this is your last week of five, and you'll try a different activity next week.

Step 2: Tuesday and Thursday: Weight Training

Repeat the plan from last week, adding weight, reaching 12 repetitions and three sets for each, and adding balance challenges. Try to go from one exercise to another without resting in between (these are called super-sets).

Step 3: Wild Card Day: New Workout

Try another new activity, or repeat your activity from last week. Also, decide what cardio interval you'll try in your next five-week session— biking, running, swimming, and so on. Then, next week, repeat this five-week plan with your new cardio interval activity.

CONGRATULATIONS! NOW DO IT AGAIN!

You did it! You worked out three to five days a week for five weeks! You've created a habit—if you try to take next week off, you'll feel anxious and uncomfortable, so don't do it! Instead, it's time to change things up. Pick a new cardio activity. If you ran for the past five weeks, now try biking or swimming or spinning for the next five. This keeps your body from reaching that plateau. By constantly doing different types of exercise, you stress different muscles, improving their tone. You also avoid repetitive use injury to your muscles, bones, ligaments, and tendons. Think of it as rotating your tires.

CHANGE IT UP

As you work through your five-week cycles, it will be tempting to go back to what you're most comfortable with—to get in a pattern of running, swimming, and biking. But I encourage you to commit to adding one entirely new exercise at least a few times a year. It's great for your confidence and for giving all your muscles a good workout. A few years ago, one of my best friends, Patti, turned me on to karate. I never would have tried this had it not been for her and her ridiculously rock-hard body (at the age of forty-five, and after three kids). I loved it! It was fun, and it was a great workout. This year, I had several patients tell me about a ballet-inspired workout called the Bar Method, based on small range of motion exercises. It turned out to be one of the best workouts I'd ever done. In five weeks, it had visibly transformed my body! The key is trying new things. Be adventurous!

 THE MAGIC OF A GOAL

At age forty-two, I'm in the best shape of my life, and it's all because of two things: I picked something new and set a goal. A friend had competed in a triathlon, and I decided I'd try it, too. I joined a training team, met new people to work out with, and discovered I loved the variety of tri-training. You're always changing your workout—swimming one day, biking the next, running the next—so you never get bored. Most of all,

I loved having a goal to work toward. It motivated me in a way I'd never experienced before with my exercise. (By the way, triathlons are becoming more and more popular, not just with elite athletes, but with ordinary people, even those who have never exercised before. To learn more about training and women's triathlons, visit www.danskintriathlon.net.)

But it's not just races that work. My friend Patti (the one with the rock-hard body) started karate because her kids were taking it. She loved the workout, but even more, she loved having a goal to shoot for. She's now working on her black belt! When we find a new activity we enjoy, we're often driven to master it. That's the magic of trying something new and setting a goal. If you can harness that magic for your health, you can transform your body inside and out.

CLOCKSTOPPING SECRETS: FIVE MORE REASONS TO LOVE EXERCISE[7]

If you find yourself avoiding your workouts, post this by your computer, your fridge, or your bed. It's not just a beautiful body you're creating with exercise, but a happier life. And nothing makes you look younger than being healthy and happy.

1. **A better mood.** Exercise releases endorphins, a substance resembling the drug morphine. This boosts your mood and immune system. Some studies suggest that exercise can help some types of depression as much as medication. If you're depressed, seek help— but talk to your doctor and therapist about how exercise can augment your treatments. See chapter 4 for more on mood management.

2. **Higher energy levels.** Being more active produces adrenaline and gives you more energy.
3. **Better sex.** Being in better shape makes you more ready and able to enjoy sex, both physically and psychologically.
4. **Better sleep.** When your body and mind are exercised regularly, your sleep can become deeper and more restful.
5. **Chronic diseases are more easily managed.** Exercise can help prevent or lessen the impact of chronic diseases, including cardiovascular disease, obesity, and depression.

CLOCKSTOPPING SECRET: FIND A YOUNGER WORKOUT BUDDY

One more exercise secret that really worked for me: Find a younger friend to exercise with. One of my favorite workout pals is twenty years younger than me—and a world-champion college ice hockey player. She's in top shape and always pushing herself—and, therefore, me. I can't match her aerobic conditioning, but I can try to approach it—and it feels great. The idea here is that if you surround yourself with younger and more fit people, some of that will rub off and motivate you as well! If you don't happen to know any world-class athletes, your teenage kids will suffice!

Weight-Training Routine

These exercises will work out some of your body's major muscles. But there are dozens of other exercises that will do similar things, and it's important not to do the same exercises month after month, year after year. Ask a trainer at your gym to show you how to use machines you're not familiar with or to suggest new exercises, or check out one of the many books, DVDs, websites, or apps demonstrating strength training moves for women.

1. PUSH-UPS

Strengthens these muscles: biceps, core/abdominals, back, and chest

Start with: 8 for beginners; 15 for advanced

Sets: Two to three sets of 8–15 repetitions ("reps"), with 1-minute rests in between (or alternate push-up sets with one of the other exercises below to get the same benefit in less time)

Target: 5 more than you think you can; you want your muscles to shake on the last few

I'm a firm believer that women should do *real* push-ups and not be brainwashed into thinking that they should do "girl" push-ups. Here's how: Place your hands about shoulders' width apart with your fingers spread wide and facing inward slightly. Extend your legs out behind you with your feet hips' width apart. Push yourself up off the floor until your arms are completely straight and a straight line is formed from your head through your body and hips to your feet. Bend your arms to ninety degrees, exhaling on the way down, and then come back up. When you go down, keep your abs sucked in, your buttocks squeezed tightly, and don't let your hips drop before your chest does. Start with just a few and slowly build up. Eventually, doing this every day, you will work up to 20, 30, 40, or more.

Balance challenge for advanced exercisers: Instead of the floor, put your hands on an extra-large exercise ball, a balance board, or even a large pillow. Adding an uneven surface makes

small muscles in your core work harder, improving the workout
without adding reps.

2. PLANK

Strengthens these muscles: core/abdominals, back, and
shoulders
Start with: 20 seconds
Target: add 15 seconds at a time, until you can do two minutes
or more

Lie on your belly on a flat, hard surface. Bend your arms inward until
you are resting on both elbows. You can clasp your hands together or
leave them apart. With one swift, unified motion, bring your entire body
off the floor, resting only on your elbows/lower arms and toes. Hold for
as many seconds as possible.

Balance Challenge 1: Rest your forearms on an exercise ball, with
your feet straight back in the same plank position you just did.
Roll the ball a few inches away from you, then back, 10 times, while
keeping your core tight.
Balance Challenge 2: While you're either on the ball or the floor,
raise one leg for 15 seconds. Then lower that and raise the other
for 15 seconds. It seems simple, but it really works your core.

3. TRICEPS KICKBACKS

Strengthens these muscles: triceps and shoulders
Start with: 8 reps
Target: 12–15 reps; add more weight when 15 seems easy

Take a 2-pound dumbbell in your right hand. Step your right leg back approximately 2 feet behind your left foot. Bend forward at your waist, keeping your back flat and your shoulders level. Extend your right arm straight back behind you until it is parallel with your torso. Making small bending movements like a hinge, bend and straighten your arm as many times as possible. Your upper arm should not move at all. When you feel like your arm is ready to fall off, congratulations! You've reached the point of muscle fatigue. Now, see if you can do five more reps! Those reps—when you don't think you can do any more, but manage to squeeze out one or two—are the ones that really make a difference. And really build your muscle fibers! Then switch sides.

4. TRICEPS DIPS

Strengthens these muscles: triceps, chest, upper back, and shoulders

Start with: 10

Target: 50

Find a chair without wheels. Position yourself sitting just on the edge. Place both hands on the edge of the chair directly under your shoulders. Scoot your butt and torso off the chair and slowly bend your arms behind you until they are at a ninety-degree angle. At this deep angle, your torso should be below the level of the chair. Bend and straighten your arms as many times as you can. The number you start with will be different for everyone, but usually fitness experts recommend starting with 10 and increasing to the point of muscle fatigue. Then do 5 more!

Balance challenge: For a better workout, put your feet on a pillow or a ball instead of the floor. This engages more tiny muscles in your core and throughout your body as you try to balance; you get a better workout in less time without increasing your reps.

5. ONE-LEG SITTING

Strengthens these muscles: gluteus maximus, thigh, hamstrings, and core/abs
Start with: 10
Target: to the point of muscle fatigue (unable to do one more)

Stand in front of a sturdy chair (don't use one with wheels). Extend one leg straight out in front of you and, keeping that leg straight, sit down using only your other leg. With your leg still extended, try to stand up, pushing off only with the other leg. If you need assistance, put light pressure on a railing next to you. Do as many as you can on one side, then switch legs.

6. TOE RAISES

Strengthens these muscles: calves
Start with: 30
Target: 2 minutes

Stand with your hand on a wall or against something sturdy. Rise up onto your tiptoes and then lower down until your heels touch the floor. Do this 30 times and build up from there to 2 minutes.

7. PELVIC TILTS

Strengthens these muscles: buttocks, quads/thighs, and
   core/abs
Start with: 1 minute
Target: 3 minutes

Lie down with your knees bent and your feet flat on the floor under your
knees. Lift and lower just your pelvis/butt from the floor as high up as
you can get it without arching your back. Squeeze your buttocks tightly
together. Hold this for 60 seconds, and gradually build up to 3 minutes.

Your Body Beautiful for Life

If you could only make a single change in your life based on this book,
I'd want it to be increasing your exercise. Every day more research
comes out showing that daily activity is the single most transformative
change you can make for your body, and that it will improve your health
in countless ways, now and for decades to come.

I know that in your thirties and forties it's almost impossible to stick
to a routine every single week. That's okay. During the weeks when you
just can't stick to it, forgive yourself and try to add *some* activity, whether
it's parking farther away, walking faster, or taking the stairs. Some exercise is better than nothing, every minute counts, and being even a
little more active, starting right now, will lay the foundation for a lifetime of good health.

3

Clockstopping Secrets
for Skin, Hair, and Beauty

A s a doctor, my first and foremost concern is *inner* beauty. I
want my patients to develop habits that will keep their bodies
healthy and strong for a lifetime. But I'm the first to admit
that I love the perks that come with these healthy habits. One of the best
side effects of creating inner beauty is the way it stops the clock on your
outer beauty, too!

What you eat, how fit your body is, and your health choices in general make an immediate, obvious impact on how your face, hair, and, to
some extent, your teeth look as you age. In fact, some experts believe
that you control a whopping 50 percent of how young you look—the
other half is determined by your genes. If your mom's skin is still flaw-
less at seventy, yours may well be, too (as long as you eat, exercise, and
sleep well). But even if your family members haven't aged so well, you
still control half of your own beauty destiny.

It's absolutely true that in your late thirties and forties you're
going to look different and older—but looking older can actually mean

looking *better*. It's a simple idea: The better you treat your body, the better your body, especially your face, skin, and hair, will treat you. If during your thirties and forties you cultivate the habits I explore in this chapter, you're going to look better ten, twenty, even thirty years from now. Some of these habits require effort and commitment; they aren't overnight remedies you can buy off the shelf. But putting the effort in during your thirties will make you look better in your forties; building these habits in your forties will pay off in your fifties and sixties. And all of them will make you more beautiful inside *and* out.

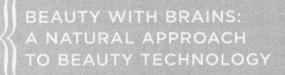

BEAUTY WITH BRAINS: A NATURAL APPROACH TO BEAUTY TECHNOLOGY

Throughout this book—and in this chapter in particular—I emphasize that everything in your body is part of a larger system. You can't simply look at your skin, your hair, and your teeth as separate, unrelated body parts: They're all part of one beautiful whole—you. So in general, I advocate using natural, organic products and approaches whenever possible, because they'll benefit your entire system. But as a Western-trained doctor, I also firmly believe in the benefits of science and technology, wisely used (sunscreen, for example). And I know that to stop the clock and improve your body and beauty, you need to use every tool in your toolbox. So my philosophy is to emphasize natural approaches first, *then* make smart decisions about higher-tech treatments. That's why I start by sharing Ayurvedic beauty advice, but then include pros and cons on beauty technologies ranging from peptides to Botox to plastic surgery. Only you can make smart decisions for yourself, based on your own physical and psychological needs—and to do that, you need all the facts.

THE BODY BEAUTIFUL PRESCRIPTION: BEAUTY

If you cultivate the following habits in your thirties and forties, you'll look younger and healthier in your later years.

1. Sleep eight hours a night.
2. Choose pure skin-care products when possible to exfoliate, moisturize, and block the sun. Use sunscreen every day, at every age, and reapply often.
3. Start using products with retinoids in your thirties.
4. If you consider Botox, plastic surgery, or other high-tech solutions, understand all the pros and cons first.
5. See your dentist three times a year for cleaning, and consider whitening your teeth.

Top-Secret Clockstopper: Sleep

Last week, Perri, a thirty-two-year-old patient, came into my office. From a gynecologic standpoint, she was fine. No problems. But she'd been sick four times in six months with various viruses and infections. She had headaches almost every day. She'd gained seven pounds in six months, her skin was breaking out, she was exercising less often, and she just didn't feel good.

"Is there something wrong with me? Can you prescribe something to help?" she asked.

I did some basic blood tests, which would take a few days to come back. Meanwhile, I told her, I did have a prescription that would help right away.

"Great," she said. "I'll do anything!"

I pulled out my prescription pad and wrote, "Sleep eight hours a night STAT."

Perri's body was sending her a message, loud and clear. Every night, she sacked out around 1 a.m. and woke at 6 a.m. Clearly, that wasn't cutting it, and her body was sending signals that it needed more rest.

Some 70 million Americans suffer from chronic sleep loss, which means that they're not getting the recommended seven to nine hours per night they need for good health. A whopping one out of three Americans sleeps six or fewer hours a night, according to the Centers for Disease Control. Sleep deprivation seems to be a national epidemic.

Even though we all do it almost every single night of our lives, sleep remains one of the most mysterious and poorly understood processes of the human body. A lack of adequate sleep has been linked to increased risks of diabetes, heart disease, obesity, depression, and high blood pressure. Studies of pilots, doctors, truck drivers, and college students have shown performance deteriorates markedly when done with little sleep. And people who wake up tired also tend to be crankier, more irritable, and less optimistic. Sleep clearly affects your body, mind, and spirit.

CLOCKSTOPPING SECRET: SLEEP MAKES YOU MORE BEAUTIFUL

In a study from Sweden, twenty-three people were photographed twice: once after a good night's sleep, then after a night of sleep deprivation. Later, the photos were shown to observers who had never met the participants. Each observer saw only one photo of each subject—before *or* after sleep deprivation, but not both. The observers who looked at the well-rested pictures judged the subjects to be healthier and more beautiful than observers who looked at the sleep-deprived set.[1]

FIVE WEEKS TO BEAUTY SLEEP

Many of my patients tell me there's absolutely no way they can sleep more than six hours a night and still get through the to-do list. I tell them that protecting and cultivating their good health needs to be at the *top* of that to-do list—and that if they start sleeping eight hours a night, they'll be amazed at how much more they get done during the day. In the end, getting enough sleep is as simple as creating new habits. But you really need to commit to making that change. Remind yourself this will make you more beautiful, healthier, and happier. Isn't that worth the effort?

Week 1: Assess Your Bedroom

I had one patient who was plagued for weeks by sleepless nights, which she attributed to stress at the new job she'd just taken in a new city. Desperate for a good night's sleep, she called a sleep clinic, got their pre-visit brochure, and followed the steps recommended before her first visit . . . including turning a fan on at night. Her very first night sleeping with the fan on solved the problem. She slept like a rock and never had to visit the sleep clinic after all. It turned out that the street traffic in her new apartment was keeping her up and she hadn't even realized it.

Similarly, simple environmental factors may be interfering with your shut-eye. So, in this first week, assess your sleeping environment.

- First, check the lighting (TV, computer, windows, streetlights). Block out all internal and external lights when you go to sleep. Even exposure to low levels of light, like that coming from electronics devices, stimulates your brain while you're sleeping, resulting in poor quality or light sleep.
- Control the climate. Sixty-five degrees Fahrenheit or thereabouts is usually best for sleeping.
- Be sure your mattress, pillows, and clothing are really comfortable.
- Think about sources of noise. Earplugs can be a great help for city dwellers, or a white-noise machine (or a fan!) can help dull surrounding sounds.
- Reform your children. Small kids can be a serious threat to sound sleep. Of course, some sleep loss is unavoidable—somebody has to soothe the nightmares. But if your children are consistently in your bed or waking you up and preventing you from getting a full night's sleep, that can be a serious problem. Talk to your pediatrician about ways to stop the night wakings so you can get the sleep you need to be a happier, healthier mom.

Week 2: Add Forty Winks a Day

This week, calculate what time you need to hit the hay if you're going to get eight hours of sleep. If you're not hitting the mark, go to bed forty minutes earlier than usual. Forty minutes represents a good chunk of time, but is usually more manageable than going to bed a whole hour earlier.

To help you make your goal, be sure to go to bed at the same time every night and wake up at the same time every day. Your body quickly establishes sleep cycles and habits. If after a week you're sleeping more, but still not eight hours, add another forty minutes every week until you're getting what you need.

Week 3: Turn Off the Tap

This week, limit your pre-bedtime beverages so you don't have to wake up to pee. Starting two hours before bedtime, don't drink anything. Also, in the late afternoons and evenings this week, make a point to avoid drinks with alcohol or caffeine, both of which are diuretics, which increase urine production, leading to a full bladder in a shorter amount of time.

Week 4: Unplug

This week, turn off the computer, the BlackBerry, and the TV thirty minutes to an hour before bedtime. Without a sensory time-out, your brain may not realize it's winding down time, no matter how exhausted your body is. If you feel you must do something before closing your eyes, lie quietly and ponder your day: Make a list of what went well, what could have gone better, and then mentally sign off until tomorrow.

Week 5: Add Some Spa Time

This week, commit to spa time before bed, even if it's only five minutes. This could be a warm bath or shower, massaging your hands and feet with lavender-infused oil, or (if you don't have a problem with night-time bathroom visits) chamomile or valerian tea. Then take five deep breaths in through your nose, out through your mouth, as soon as you get in bed. Even a few minutes of a focused, relaxing ritual can make it easier to fall asleep.

After committing to a new, improved sleep routine for five weeks, assess what worked for you and what didn't. If you're still having trouble, read on to the section about insomnia and sleep changes over time, and talk with your doctor. You deserve your beauty sleep!

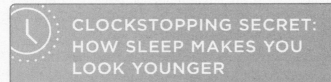

CLOCKSTOPPING SECRET: HOW SLEEP MAKES YOU LOOK YOUNGER

Studies show that consistently getting a good night's sleep:

- may lessen appearance of dark circles under your eyes.
- reduces skin changes caused by dehydration.
- helps cellular repair and regeneration.
- improves mood. It may sound trite, but it's true. When you're happier, you look younger, more relaxed, and more beautiful.

SLEEP AS WE AGE

When I was in college, I bartended three nights a week, came home at 5 a.m., and went to class by 10 a.m. As an obstetrician, I spent endless nights awake with patients in labor, then came home, showered, changed, and went back to work a "normal" day (although, trust me, no day feels normal when you've been up all night). I thought my body could take it, but it never felt great. Now, at forty-two, I make it a priority to sleep eight to nine hours a night, even if that means skipping a night with my friends or watching my favorite hockey team. And I promise you, I feel better than I did in my twenties or thirties.

Our sleep needs change as we age:[2]

- Newborn baby: 16–18 hours a day
- Ages 1–12: 13–14 hours a day
- Teenagers: 9–11 hours a day
- Adults: 8–9 hours a day

While "adults" are usually lumped into one category, researchers at Cornell University have found that as people get older, they tend to sleep for shorter periods of time.[3] You may find your sleep quality diminishes as you get close to fifty; you may awaken several times a night or find it harder to fall asleep in the first place.

What's important here is to understand that when it comes to sleep, one size does not fit all. Your sleep needs, patterns, and habits will change as you age, and they're the first thing you should look at when you're worried about your energy levels or overall health. If you find your sleep quality declines as you age, it's more important than ever that you practice good sleep habits, and talk to your doctor if sleep problems continue. Your mother was right: You need your rest—at *any* age.

UP ALL NIGHT: INSOMNIA

If you've ever suffered from insomnia for more than a day or two, you know how sleep becomes a sort of holy grail. You think about it all day, and worry you won't sleep at night (and worrying about not sleeping can actually keep you up).

Insomnia is the inability to fall asleep or stay asleep as long as you want or need to. Lonely as it feels in the wee hours, remember that you're not alone. In fact, the National Institutes of Health estimate that one in three Americans suffer occasional insomnia, and 10 percent report chronic insomnia, where they can't fall asleep or stay asleep for at least three nights a week, for more than a month.[4] Women seem to be particularly prone to sleep problems and disturbances. In one poll, some 63 percent of women reported occasional symptoms of insomnia, compared with 54 percent of men.[5]

When patients speak to me about insomnia, I first look for a medical or medicinal cause. A host of medical problems can disrupt sleep. Depression, sinus problems, back or neck pain, cardiac disease, respiratory conditions such as coughing or sleep apnea, heartburn or GERD (reflux), bowel or bladder issues, hormonal changes, or even skin conditions such as unremitting itching can all interfere with sleep. Ironically, so can many of the medications used to treat these ailments. Fortunately, once you realize there's a medical cause for your insomnia, it's usually easy to solve the sleep problem.

When there's no obvious medical reason, the next step is to try safe, effective treatments. With sleep problems, the simplest effective solution is always the best. I advise my patients to start with natural, environmental, and behavioral changes before trying any kind of sleep aid—even so-called p.m. pain relievers sold over the counter. Natural remedies usually have no major downsides, and may be less likely to have side effects or interactions with other medications.

If my patients try following my Body Beautiful sleep plan but see no improvement, I may recommend a sleep aid for short-term use. I usually start by recommending mild, over-the-counter remedies, like melatonin, a chemical released in your brain in response to darkness, telling us it's time to go to sleep. Melatonin is a natural substance, available in supplemental form over the counter. Some people feel it works well, though its effect may take weeks before it is noticed. Like any supplement, do not assume more is better: Take only what is recommended on the label. If, after four weeks, you don't notice any improvement, stop taking it.

Another over-the-counter remedy I mentioned above are the pain relievers labeled "p.m." These contain Benadryl, a sedative that may help you fall asleep, but won't necessarily help you stay in a deep, restorative, REM phase of sleep.

Prescription sleep aids include relaxants or sedatives (such as Valium or Xanax) and so-called hypnotics (like Ambien). This last category works via the central nervous system through mechanisms that are not well understood. Any of these medicines can be very helpful and effective for a short period. But I will only prescribe them for short-term use—either once or twice a week or, if my patient is going through a specific, temporary period of high stress, nightly for no more than a few weeks.

I'm very careful to limit the time my patients can take prescription sleep aids, because it's easy to become dependent on them. Even without being physically addicted, you can become psychologically dependent on a sleep aid, believing you need them to fall asleep (when you really don't). Psychological dependence is a perfect example of how something helpful and therapeutic can become problematic and dangerous if not taken properly. If you find that you are needing more of a prescription medication to get a good night's rest or, even worse, are combining multiple sleep medications, speak to your doctor immediately. Accidental overdose or drug dependence can happen to anyone.

If you're considering any prescription sleep aid, be sure to talk over the pros and cons with your doctor and understand how to use it safely. Use it to get the sleep you need in the short term, while cultivating good sleep habits that keep you well rested for the rest of your life.

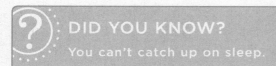

DID YOU KNOW?
You can't catch up on sleep.

If you lose sleep one night, don't try to make up for it on the weekend. Turns out you can't really catch up on sleep. Instead, stick to your bedtime schedule as if you were Cinderella at the ball.

Skin-Deep: Clockstopping Secrets for Radiant Skin

A good night's sleep does wonders for your skin, but time still takes its toll. As you age, the surface layer of your skin, called the epidermis, becomes more fragile and less resilient. It doesn't repair damage (from sunburn, late nights, or unhealthy foods) as quickly as it once did. Beneath the epidermis, the inner layer, called the dermis, begins losing the protein and collagen fibers that keep it plump. This causes skin to sag. In addition, the machinery in our skin, like the sweat glands we cursed in our teens for causing zits, becomes less active, reducing moisture in our skin. Meanwhile, fibers under the skin, called elastin, are destroyed over time by sun, smoking, and other factors, resulting in wrinkles.

You can't replace or restore elastin, but you can postpone its loss, improve your complexion, and slow the aging process in several ways: by controlling your environment and your diet, learning about alternative beauty treatments, and, of course, cosmetic dermatology treatments. Each of these has its own advantages and drawbacks. Here's what you need to know to make your own smart decisions.

THE ENVIRONMENT

To keep your skin looking young and fresh forever, the best thing you could do would be to live in a windowless basement. Barring that, you could start noticing how much sun you get every day, even on a cloudy day. You might not think you're in the sun much, but start adding up the time you spend driving your car, walking to the mailbox, running errands, walking the dog, even sitting near windows. It all takes its toll. Some dermatologists believe that a whopping 80 percent of all sun exposure comes not from sitting at the beach but from many short stints in the sun.

That's why it's absolutely vital to use a moisturizer with a sun protection factor (SPF) every day, and to reapply it several times during the day. Look for an SPF factor of at least 30, regardless of your skin type, but even higher if you're fair-skinned. Make sure the product you choose has both UVB and UVA protection. This will block out both UVB, or ultraviolet, rays causing sunburn and UVA rays, which contribute to wrinkles. Both types cause skin cancer as well. Typically, products that have both UVA and UVB protection contain the ingredients avobenzone, titanium dioxide, or basic zinc oxide.

CLOCKSTOPPING SECRET: REAPPLY SUNSCREEN TO YOUR FACE DURING THE DAY

Applying sunscreen in the morning is only your first step in protecting yourself from the sun. Here's what you need to do every day to keep your skin young.

- Apply lotion with SPF to your face every day as soon as you brush your teeth.
- Apply more sunscreen at least twenty minutes before going outside.
- Reapply sunscreen if you're going outside, and reapply every two to four hours until you go indoors.
- Reapply after sweating or swimming.
- If you're applying it to your entire body, use about as much sunscreen as would fill a shot glass.
- Discard sunscreen every six months, because it expires.

CLOCKSTOPPING SECRET:
USE RETINOIDS AFTER THIRTY

Retinoids are a class of skin creams made of a vitamin A derivative. When converted to their active form, called retinoic acid, this substance has powerful and positive effects on the skin. Retinoic acid works inside the nucleus of the cell to activate genes. These genes control a variety of functions, including those that govern how skin cells divide, as well as how they shed and renew themselves. These genes also stimulate collagen production, and have exfoliating and anti-inflammatory actions. Many products contain retinol or retinoids, but the strongest concentrations are only available by prescription. You might start with an over-the-counter product containing retinol and use it two or three times a week; it may take twelve weeks to see a difference. For a faster or more powerful effect, ask a dermatologist to prescribe a stronger retinoid.

Some people have some initial sensitivity to these creams or lotions, but usually this goes away as your skin adjusts to the treatment. Using a retinoid every other night or nightly can have amazing effects on your skin, although some changes take months to appear. Not only can retinoids make you look younger and your skin more vibrant, but use of products containing retinoids can delay skin aging in the first place. Talk to your dermatologist about whether a prescription-strength retinoid cream is right for you. I use one every night and can see a huge improvement in my skin. It almost makes those years of being a lifeguard disappear!.

CLOCKSTOPPING SECRET: OMEGA-3 FATTY
ACIDS AND ANTIOXIDANTS

It's absolutely no surprise that healthier eating gives you younger-looking skin. Studies have shown that foods high in omega-3 fatty acids tend to be good for the skin because they can reduce inflammation, which makes your skin look more irritated, less radiant, and, frankly, older. Fortunately, it's a delicious prescription. Foods high in omega-3 fatty acids include salmon, avocado, and nuts.

Foods containing antioxidants can also help keep your skin looking younger by reducing the impact of day-to-day skin stress. Just living on planet Earth exposes your skin cells to a constant assault from the sun, pollution, bacteria, and viruses. The result is oxidative stress, a condition where your skin becomes less adept at healing itself. Fortunately, foods high in antioxidants, including blueberries, pomegranates, tart cherries, and dark chocolate, can repair damage from oxidation and rejuvenate your cells. And guess what? If you follow my Five-Day/Two-Day Plan (see chapter 1), you'll automatically get more antioxidants through those unlimited amounts of fruits and veggies you can eat. What a coincidence!

Meanwhile, cut back on other foods that cause cellular inflammation. Specifically, cut back on white bread, white sugar, potatoes, and processed foods—anything high in simple carbohydrates and refined sugar. Also avoid greasy, fried food—the extra oil isn't helping lubricate your skin, trust me.[6] And again—what do you know! The Five-Day/Two-Day Plan will help cut these from your diet, too.

CLOCKSTOPPING SECRET: CHANGE YOUR SKIN PRODUCTS AS YOU AGE

One size does *not* fit all when it comes to skin care. Your skin changes every decade, and so should your skin-care products. Women over thirty should use products with an alpha hydroxy or retinol ingredient, and women of all ages should use products with peptides as ingredients.

- **For All Ages:** Use sunscreen daily, and look for age-appropriate skin-care products. Many manufacturers, including Olay and Aveeno, formulate product lines for specific age groups. Usually, the manufacturer's website can tell you which line is right for you.
- **Daily Skin Routine for Your Thirties:** Use products with retinoids and alpha hydroxy several times a week to reverse effects of aging and sun damage. (You don't have to use expensive products to get alpha hydroxy; see the mask I recommend below!)
- **Daily Skin Routine for Your Forties:** Continue using products with retinoids, and add a product with peptides, the latest technology in delivering nutrients to your skin cells. Consider a daily aspirin, if your doctor says it's okay (see the "Acids and Aspirin" section to find out why).

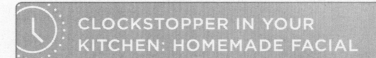

CLOCKSTOPPER IN YOUR KITCHEN: HOMEMADE FACIAL

I like to mix my own all-natural mask at home by combining sugar, honey, milk, and oatmeal. I mix it all up in a bowl and rub it all over my face. I leave it on for approximately fifteen minutes, once a week.

Acids and Aspirin

Alpha and beta hydroxy acids are found in sugar cane, milk, apples, citrus, and wine, and reduce fine lines and wrinkles. They work as exfoliants, chemically removing the surface layer of dead skin cells, allowing newer, fresher cells to take their place. This might improve the surface texture or discoloration of your skin, including sun spots or freckles, although you might not see any results for several months. These acids are found in many moisturizers—but, as I point out above, you can make your own hydroxy acid masks by applying milk and certain fruits, like citrus fruits or banana, as a facial mask.

One everyday source of beta hydroxy acid is derived from aspirin, so recently some skin-care experts have started to recommend low-dose aspirin as a way to reduce wrinkling from the inside out. So far, the jury is out: Research is ongoing to see if aspirin taken orally can help wrinkles. With no clear answers to this controversial question, it doesn't make sense to start popping baby aspirin daily until you talk to your doctor. Even in low doses, aspirin can increase the risk of internal bleeding, so some people shouldn't take aspirin at all. Then again, if your doctor says it won't hurt, there's some chance it might help. I'm not against taking an aspirin a day as long as you have medical approval, but I'm not yet convinced it will help your face.

CLOCKSTOPPING SECRET: PEPTIDES

An exciting new technological advance in skin care may help you look younger: bioactive peptides. Hang on for a little chemistry here.

Peptides are chains of amino acids. Think of them as tiny building blocks of protein molecules, including collagen, one of the most important types of protein in your skin. These peptides are busy structures. They attach to various receptors within our skin cells. Receptors are like loading docks: They're places where substances and messages are delivered from one cell to another. When peptides "dock" at a receptor, they affect a wide variety of processes, including inflammation, cell repair, and new protein production. Meanwhile, peptides are so small that they can easily penetrate the deeper layers of the skin, delivering substances like antioxidants to these hard-to-reach layers. In addition, when other skin cells start seeing lots of peptides around, they act as if the skin has been damaged and start making more collagen in a type of repair mechanism. All this is great news for aging skin. Even better news is the fact that scientists have recently started altering peptide chains so they instruct cells to carry out very specific tasks (like reducing inflammation or making more collagen). In doing this, these compounds can be more powerful, more easily absorbed into the skin, and more effective at their tasks.

Bioactive peptides are rapidly becoming the new cutting-edge ingredients, already available in some skin-care products. You'll see more of these in the future. Look for products with the ugly-sounding but highly effective ingredients palmitoyl pentapeptide, oligopeptide, copper peptide, or copper gluconate. In these products, bioactive peptides will be able to trigger more collagen production (leading to firmer skin) and reduce harmful effects of toxins and inflammation (which will delay the appearance of aging). Though research is ongoing, bioactive peptides appear to be destined to occupy a key role in skin care, along with anti-inflammatories and antioxidants.[7]

CLOCKSTOPPER AU NATUREL: THE AYURVEDIC ALTERNATIVE

About ten years ago, I read *Absolute Beauty* by Dr. Pratima Raichur, a fascinating book about Ayurveda, the eastern Indian philosophy of health and wellness. Not long afterward, I visited her skin-care spa in New York and had the good fortune to meet her in person. She's been a friend and beauty inspiration ever since. Now seventy, Pratima looks fifty and emits an aura of health, wellness, and inner beauty. She's taught me a great deal about the Ayurvedic approach to wellness, much of which I've incorporated into my practice with my patients. In my own life, I've followed her principles, and I honestly think my skin has improved a great deal. That's why, with her blessings, I have to share some of Pratima's secrets with you.

Ayurvedic Secret 1: If it's not pure enough to eat, don't use it on your face.

Skin is the body's largest organ. It can absorb medications and other substances into the bloodstream, so we should be as attentive to what we put on our skin as what we put into our mouths. If you look at the active and inactive ingredients in many popular skin-care products, you may be shocked to learn that several of them are on the FDA's list of known or suspected human carcinogens. Among those are innocent-sounding substances like mineral oil, BHA, and BHT, all on the list of known or suspected cancer-causing agents. Since we already have plenty of daily exposure to suspected carcinogens in our environment, I prefer not to put any additional ones on my skin. It's easy—*and cheap*—to substitute natural and inexpensive alternatives for these potentially dangerous substances. See the box called "Natural Beauty" for suggestions.

On the other hand, if you're very concerned about wrinkles and very interested in the latest science, all my advice on peptides and retinoids stands. What would be ideal would be organic versions of these advanced treatments, guaranteeing they don't contain some of the substances I name above. But even lacking that, it's not an either/or decision. You can still choose natural treatments when possible (say, my kitchen facial now and then, together with your daily moisturizer with bioactive peptides and SPF). As always, you need to make your own choices about what's best for your values, your lifestyle, and your goals for your personal appearance.

NATURAL BEAUTY

For a natural approach to moisturizing, exfoliating, and skin care, try these:

For body moisturizer: Use sunflower or safflower oil from the grocery store. I use this on myself and my children regularly, adding a few drops of lavender oil for an aromatherapy boost.

For cleanser: Mix almond meal, dry milk, and sugar into a paste and apply to dry skin.

For exfoliator: Mix sugar with a few drops of milk and honey. Use as a facial scrub.

For breakouts: Mix ½ teaspoon crushed cumin seed, 1 teaspoon coriander, and a few drops of water to form a paste. Leave on for thirty minutes, then rinse. Apply twice a week.

Ayurvedic Secret 2: Exfoliate (Especially After Thirty)

Using a natural sugar scrub, make this weekly ritual a part of your skin-care routine. As your skin becomes less efficient at cell turnover, the surface layer of your skin can appear dull. Gently removing those dead skin cells will bring a youthful glow to your skin. Pratima recommends making a mask out of banana or avocado pulp and letting it sit on your face for fifteen minutes with your legs raised to increase blood flow to the head. Exfoliation is important after age thirty and into the forties, as skin becomes more dry.

Ayurvedic Secret 3: Hydrate and Moisturize Aggressively from Both the Inside and the Outside (Especially After Forty)

Increase your intake of water to the point that your urine is clear or light yellow. Take 1,000 mg of an omega-3 fatty acid supplement daily (which you're already doing, if you're following the advice in chapter 1), and step up your facial moisturizing routine to include both morning and evening, if you don't do that already. Use a heavier moisturizer at night to seal in moisture while you're sleeping.

Ayurvedic Secret 4: Exercise More (Especially Near and After Fifty-Something)

Increasing your physical exercise will increase blood flow to the face, enhancing your skin's natural color and glow and helping to revive all the cells that may be lying down on the job of moisturizing your skin. At least thirty minutes of vigorous exercise five times a week will work wonders for your complexion. (Sex counts!)

A LITTLE HELP, HERE? BOTOX, FILLERS, AND LASER RESURFACING

At the other end of the spectrum, away from the all-natural approach, is technology. I'm not averse to using both approaches; again, this isn't an either/or decision. I believe in trying natural remedies and treatments and assessing whether they work for your skin and your personal appearance goals. But every body is different, and all the sunscreen, blueberries, and hydration in the world can't let us keep our dewy young complexion forever. Many of my patients turn to skin-care treatments by dermatologists. I can't tell them whether it's right or wrong to use Botox; that's not my job. Instead, the most important thing I can do is encourage them to understand all the pros and cons of every treatment they consider.

Dermatologist 101: Finding the Right Doctor

First, make sure your skin doctor *is* a doctor—and a trustworthy one. These days, plenty of people who aren't M.D.s, including dentists, "anti-aging specialists" (not an accredited medical specialty, by the way), even "medical day spas" offer Botox injections and other treatments. But you don't want just anyone sticking a needle in your face, even if he or she is a doctor. Instead, find a dermatologist or plastic surgeon with specialized training in the face, skin, and facial nerves. These doctors are better equipped than other doctors (and certainly better than nondoctors!) to handle potential complications that may arise after injections. Word of mouth is often the best way to find a good dermatologist. If you know someone who looks great, don't hesitate to ask her if she has a dermatologist she likes.

You'll know you've found the right doctor if he or she is careful to explain the pros and cons of treatments like those I describe in this section. If he or she advises you not to proceed with a treatment, listen and ask questions. That may be the sign of a doctor you can trust for a long time to come. In medicine, we often say the best surgeon is the one who knows when *not* to cut. The same principle applies to dermatologists. Your doctor may feel you're not the best candidate for these treatments, or even that you don't need them. Listening to his or her advice may be the best way to end up with your most beautiful face, one that moves and looks like the real *you*—not like a sculpture.

When shopping for a doctor:

- seek out a board-certified dermatologist or plastic surgeon for the procedure you're considering.

- whether you're interested in Botox, injectable fillers, or a face-lift, find someone who performs a whole lot of these procedures every day. You want someone who can do this in her sleep with her hands tied behind her back. You don't want your face to be someone else's training ground.
- ask to see before and after pictures of real patients! Any reputable plastic surgeon or cosmetic dermatologist will have these photos and will be happy to show them to you.

BOTOX

Botox, a protein produced by the bacterium *Clostridium botulinum*, is one of the most lethal neurotoxins in existence—and, when injected, it's the single most common cosmetic procedure performed in the United States.[8] In 2010 alone, some 2.4 million procedures were performed.

Botox works to reduce or prevent the appearance of wrinkles by paralyzing the facial muscles so that the skin overlying those muscles looks smooth. Like all treatments, it has its pros and cons.

PROS
- Smooth, less wrinkled appearance
- Effects last three to four months
- Quick, cheap, and reversible (the effects eventually wear off)

CONS
- Possible bruising
- Overparalysis, causing eyelid drooping, brow sagging, or a lack of animation. These can affect areas near the injection site, making your face look frozen or masklike, or can result in an uneven appearance if the injections are not done by a skilled physician.

INJECTABLE FILLERS

Officially called soft tissue augmentation, injectable fillers are substances injected into skin lines to plump up sagging and creasing areas. Fillers work by physically replacing the volume that used to be in certain areas with a type of hyaluronic acid (a component of skin). In general, good candidates for fillers include people who are generally healthy, do not smoke, and have realistic goals for their appearance. (This means someone who wants to look like herself, only slightly younger, *not* someone my mother's age who wants to look like Angelina Jolie!) The injection of fillers is one of the top five cosmetic procedures performed in the United States every year, with 80 percent of patients being over forty years of age.

PROS
- Can reduce the appearance of sagging and wrinkles
- Most are temporary, so if you don't like the result, all you have to do is wait or have them removed with a type of antidote substance that counteracts the filler

CONS
Most potential complications are rare and not serious. They include:

- Bruising at the injection site
- Hardening of the substance leading to a ropy texture or appearance
- Allergic reaction to the substance
- Asymmetric appearance
- Unsatisfactory cosmetic results (in other words, you don't look like you'd hoped)

LASER RESURFACING

Full disclosure: I'm a fan of laser resurfacing. My early years as a freckle-faced lifeguard have come back to bite me, even though I became a sunscreen devotee in my early thirties (thank goodness!).

In general, laser treatments cause a mild thermal injury in the dermis (the layer beneath the surface of your skin), which causes a mild degree of scarring and an increase in collagen production along with a rejuvenation of the surface of skin cells. There are a variety of laser treatments ranging in cost and recovery time. Most treatments take approximately thirty to forty minutes. You may require several treatments to reach your desired results. Recovery can take a few hours or a few weeks, depending on the type of laser used.

PROS
- Results can be dramatic, including improved surface texture of skin, reduced appearance of fine wrinkles, and reduced discoloration

CONS
- Redness, scarring, and changes in color of skin (either lighter or darker)
- A moderate degree of pain
- Can worsen chronic skin conditions like acne or rosacea

Other procedures, such as chemical peels and dermabrasion, work similarly to laser resurfacing, but differ in the amount of recovery time and the depth in the skin reached by each procedure.

THE KINDEST CUT: IS COSMETIC SURGERY RIGHT FOR YOU?

I'm lucky to have a plastic surgeon for a brother. He lets me ask all kinds of juicy questions, the kinds of things most of us are dying to know but wouldn't admit. Here's what I've learned:

1. **Should you even consider plastic surgery?**

   This is a very personal and individual question. Some people feel comfortable aging naturally, and feel good about however they look. Others feel that in principle, there's no difference between wearing makeup, coloring their hair, and having a face-lift. In this line of thinking, all beauty treatments lie along a spectrum, with plastic surgery at one extreme. If you're considering plastic surgery, remember, it's not about whether your spouse approves, whether your friends approve, or whether your coworkers approve. It's whether *you* approve—*after* you've gathered all the facts.

   Sensible reasons for plastic surgery include dissatisfaction with the signs of aging that you see and a desire to look like yourself, only younger (and again, not like Angelina Jolie).

   But if you want plastic surgery because you want to look completely different, because you hate everything about yourself, or because you're depressed, cosmetic surgery will not help you. The process won't solve your problems and you won't be happy with the results. A responsible physician can identify patients like this a mile away and will not treat them.

2. **What's the best age and timing for cosmetic surgery?**

   That depends on your goals. Early face-lifts (in the thirties, forties, and fifties) can yield great results in the right patients. Often, the changes can be subtle and long-lasting. Subtle changes usually lead to great patient satisfaction, compared with radical changes that may accompany procedures performed after years of aging. So if you think a face-lift is in your future, you might consider checking in with a surgeon earlier than you'd planned.

Other factors to consider include recovery time and other medical conditions. The best cosmetic surgery patient is a nonsmoker in excellent physical health. Though everyone heals at different rates, most women will heal from a face-lift in approximately three weeks. That said, *all* surgical procedures carry some risk, including the risk of serious complications (heart attack, allergic reaction, infection, and even death). This makes the selection of the appropriate surgeon and surgical setting critically important.

3. **How do you choose a surgeon?**

As with any surgery, you want a doctor who does hundreds of the specific surgery you want, somebody who's seen it all and can practically do it in his or her sleep. Okay, I'm exaggerating. But this is your *face* we're talking about here, and experience counts. While all plastic surgeons are extensively trained in face-lifts, not all are experts in this procedure. Some plastic surgeons specialize in breast surgery, others in noses, others in complex reconstruction after trauma or cancer treatments, and still others in surgery of the face. Ask a lot of people, including friends and doctors you know. Then interview your prospective surgeons. Ask how many face-lifts he or she does each year. Look for someone who does fifty or more per year.

4. **What exactly do you need, anyway?**

The best way to answer this question is to ask several different surgeons. They may give you several different approaches and recommendations. My brother says that, in general, plastic surgeons think of the face as having three zones: upper, middle, and lower.

Often, they all need to be corrected for the best results. A change in one area may call for a change in another. Beware of the surgeon who tells you they will just do a brow lift, when you may be more satisfied having other areas adjusted as well. Rarely does one part of your body age in isolation. So think about all three zones, and how the others will look if you alter one.

Tress Distress:
Caring for Your Hair

Let's face it. We never have the hair we want. If it's curly, we want it straight, and vice versa. Alas, as our hormones change in our thirties, forties, and fifties, our tress distress may only increase. At least once a week, a patient comes into my office with complaints about her hair— too much body hair, thinning hair on her head, a drier, frizzier texture. Here's what's happening up on your head as you age.

Hair is mostly made up of a protein called keratin. It grows from follicles in the dermis, which are always in one of three stages of their life cycle. Anagen, the growth stage, lasting two to six years, where hair grows about a half inch per month; catagen, the transition stage after active growth, lasting about two to three weeks; and telogen, a resting phase of about one hundred days. At any given time, about 10–15 percent of our hair follicles are in the resting stage. As you age, this process continues, but the quality of your hair may change.

HAIR IN YOUR THIRTIES

In your thirties, your hair is likely to be similar to your hair early in your life. But some women in their thirties experience excess hair growth on their bodies. Some conditions, like polycystic ovarian syndrome (PCOS), may lead to high testosterone levels, producing excessive growth of hair over the entire body, especially the face (chin, cheeks, or upper lip), chest, abdomen between the belly button and pubic bone, and the lower back. If you notice more hair than normal in these locations, see your doctor. He or she may want to do some simple blood tests to check for hormonal imbalances. There are many ways to treat unwanted hair, including waxing, shaving, electrolysis, and laser treatments. Depending on your budget, these methods are all safe and effective.

HAIR DURING AND AFTER PREGNANCY

While pregnant, many women notice their hair grows faster and thicker, and enjoy the best hair days of their lives.

If only it lasted! But by six months after delivery, the reverse is happening. Lots of hair starts to fall out . . . and the remaining hair may be thinner than it was before pregnancy. This sudden loss of hair has its own scary-sounding name: telogen effluvium. Fortunately, it's only temporary. Most of the hair that falls out postpartum enters a growth phase again around six months after it falls out. As stressful as this is, rest assured that your hair will return to normal soon.

HAIR IN YOUR FORTIES

In your forties, you may notice that your hair appears thinner or drier than it did in your thirties. This might signal decreasing estrogen, or it could be caused by styling products or hair treatments. Adjusting your hair routine may help—lay off the spray and blow-dryer for a week or so and see if things improve. If not, a dermatologist can weigh in and tell you if there's a physical reason for the dryness.

CLOCKSTOPPING SECRET: YOUNGER-LOOKING HAIR

You don't need to invest a lot in fancy hair moisturizers to revitalize your hair. Try butter or olive oil. No kidding. Once a week (usually on the weekend), I massage oil into my hair after a shower and keep my hair in a ponytail under a hat all day. It ain't pretty, but it really works well to replace moisture. The hair shaft can and does absorb oils, just as it absorbs chlorine and bleach. Coating the outside of the hair shaft is one way to protect its color and texture.

Another measure that may (or may not) help is taking biotin supplements. Biotin is a water-soluble vitamin in the B family, found in cooked eggs, avocado, wheat bran products, and other foods. Biotin deficiency (which is quite rare) can cause hair loss, so some dermatologists feel the reverse may also be true—that biotin supplements can improve hair health within the shaft. However, the data supporting these benefits are controversial. My own advice is that biotin might not help, but because it's water-soluble, you won't overdose, so there's no harm in taking one supplement a day and seeing if it makes a difference.

STRAIGHT TALK: THE DANGERS OF BRAZILIAN BLOWOUTS

Recently, the trend of the Brazilian blowout has swept the country, catching on with women in search of sleek, shiny, and blessedly low-maintenance hair. This procedure, and those similar to it, uses a protein-enhanced solution that is applied to the hair and then "sealed in" using the high and intense heat of a blow-dryer and/or flatiron. In late 2010, there were multiple reports of hair stylists and customers becoming sick with complaints of burning eyes, headaches, dizziness, and even breathing problems. After investigation by several states' Occupational Safety and Health Administrations, many of these products were found to contain significant levels of formaldehyde, despite being labeled as formaldehyde-free! While small levels of this chemical are present in the air and other products, exposure to higher levels may cause certain types of cancer. Bottom line: Don't risk your health for gorgeous hair! Ask your salon to show you the labels on the products they are using. If they contain formaldehyde, don't use them. If you feel sick during a blowout, stop and get some fresh air immediately. Short-term exposure to this chemical won't make you sick, but if you get this treatment frequently, the health risks may really add up.

Long in the Tooth

Here's an aspect of aging that takes almost everyone by surprise: Your teeth change. They get darker and duller over time, as years of coffee, soda, red wine, or cigarettes start to catch up with us. At the same time, as you age, hormonal changes may decrease the amount of saliva your mouth produces, which can increase plaque buildup. When that happens, your teeth stain more easily, because plaque (bacteria covering the teeth, especially at the base near the gum) gives food and liquids something to grab on to. After three or four decades of chewing, tearing, and possibly grinding at night or during the day (called bruxism), they lose some of their resiliency. Finally, fillings that we got earlier in our lives tend to become loose or crack; when that happens, bacteria and plaque can work their way into crevices and set off a domino effect of more decay.

You may also notice your teeth feeling uncomfortable or your bite changing. As you age, teeth often shift position within the jaw. The front teeth tend to get more crowded. Meanwhile, gum disease can create gaps or spaces between teeth.

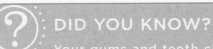

DID YOU KNOW?

Your gums and teeth change with time.

Aging gums may:
- recede, bleed, get inflamed, or get periodontal disease.
- experience more plaque due to a decrease in the mouth's saliva production.
- bleed more in response to hormonal changes, including menopause, but also birth control pills or pregnancy.

Aging teeth may:
- change in color, becoming darker and less bright.
- lose resiliency.
- dull due to chewing and grinding.
- experience more plaque and decay.
- shift in position (producing gaps or crowding).

YOUNG GUMS

While the most obvious changes you see may be in your tooth color, a far more serious problem may be taking place in your gums. As we age, our gums can become dry, start to recede, and become more susceptible to inflammation. Some age-related hormonal changes increase your risk of periodontal disease (PD), also known as gum disease. It's a condition that causes inflammation affecting gum tissue, bones, and ligaments of the mouth. Overall, experts estimate that some 75 percent of adults have PD, and most don't have any idea that they have it! In fact, it may be the most common inflammatory condition affecting humans. It creeps up on people, often with no symptoms whatsoever, until the dentist announces its presence. And it's a major cause of loss of bone density in the jawbones that hold your teeth in place.

Periodontal disease is bad news: Untreated, it leads to gum loss and eventually tooth loss. Unfortunately, the gums don't always show obvious signs of PD. As the gums recede, bone loss can occur, but the two processes don't always go hand in hand. Sometimes the gums seem to stay put, but "pockets" form beneath them where plaque and bacteria build up, which only worsens the problem. And that's just what goes on in your mouth. PD has also been linked to preterm labor in pregnant women as well as to heart disease. The treatments are no fun, either. They include scaling and root planing (scraping the hardened plaque, called tartar, from the tooth and roots) or gum surgery. Ouch!

Risk Factors for Periodontal Disease

Family history/genetics
Not brushing or flossing
Diets high in sugar or acids
Smoking or tobacco exposure
Bad dental work or poorly configured fillings
Changes in oral bone structure or anatomy
Hormonal changes

WATCH YOUR MOUTH!
ORAL HEALTH AS YOU AGE

In your thirties and forties: Your gums may bleed more right before your period. The theory is that as your progesterone levels change right before your period, blood vessels in your gums tend to widen or stretch and bleed more easily when you brush. Birth control pills containing a synthetic progesterone hormone called desogestrel can also lead to increased risk of periodontal disease.

When you're pregnant: You may experience more gum inflammation and bleeding, again due to changing levels of progesterone in your blood. Oral hygiene is even more important when you're pregnant, because PD has been linked to higher risks of preterm labor and delivery.

In your late forties and fifties: As you approach menopause, declining levels of estrogen can lead to bone loss, which affects the jaw as well as the teeth. If you notice any changes in your mouth in terms of gums and their appearance, the amount of saliva in your mouth, visible sores, or increase in bleeding, see your dentist soon.

FLOSS ON!

All this may sound like bad news. But things are a lot better today than for most of human history, when most people lost their teeth in old age. The big lesson: There's a lot you can do to prevent or slow the aging process in your mouth.

The easiest, best things you can do are brush properly, floss every day, and befriend your dentist: You should have your teeth cleaned two or three times a year.

Keeping Your Teeth Young

- Floss religiously. Dentists suggest wrapping the floss around the base of each tooth in an up-and-down and circular manner. Some people avoid flossing because their gums bleed or, even worse, the floss can unearth disgusting smells! But when those things happen, you know you're doing something right. You've found bacteria and you're getting rid of it. So floss on!
- Brush morning, noon, and night. Most of us brush in the morning and at bedtime, but brushing after meals during the day can make

a big difference. Many dentists recommend an electric toothbrush, which can help remove more plaque than regular toothbrushes. Whatever brush you use, you should replace it (or the head, if it's an electric toothbrush) every one to three months.

- Use a toothpaste that is approved by the American Dental Association, and look for those with fluoride and triclosan (an antibacterial substance than can help reduce mild gum inflammation).

- Use a mouthwash: The liquid can get into nooks and crannies that your toothbrush can't. Your dentist can write you a prescription for a mouthwash made of chlorhexidine, which kills bacteria and can reduce plaque by 30 to 45 percent.

CLOCKSTOPPING SECRET: WHITER AND BRIGHTER

One of the simplest things you can do to look younger and more vibrant is to whiten your teeth. It's easy to do, approved by the American Dental Association, and you can choose from lots of methods, ranging from over-the-counter solutions to in-office procedures. Whitening procedures probably won't return your teeth to the luminous whiteness of childhood, and not all stains respond to bleaching (especially darkening caused by the antibiotic tetracycline), but they can lighten your teeth by several shades. It's a subtle change that can make a big difference in your appearance. Before you start on a whitening project, though, see your dentist and make sure your gums and teeth are in good shape.

There aren't many risks, but they include discomfort due to sensitivity of teeth to the brightening chemicals or a chemical burn to the gums from the bleaching products. Both are temporary and tend to resolve within days.

MORE TREATMENTS FOR
A BRIGHTER SMILE

Veneers

If your teeth are cracked, chipped, badly stained, or irregular in size or shape, veneers may be the answer. Dental veneers are wafers of porcelain or resin that bond to your teeth. After a general consultation, your dentist makes molds of your teeth to form the custom-made veneers, which usually take three visits to apply.

> Pros: Veneers can make a huge difference in your appearance.
> Cons: Veneers can be expensive. And, although technically they're permanent, they may need to be replaced in ten years or so.

Embracing Braces

You've probably noticed that braces aren't just for teenagers anymore. A growing number of adults are having their teeth straightened, and some of today's braces barely show. If you're self-conscious about your teeth, consult with an orthodontist. The consultation will include X-rays; any cavities or gum disease have to be treated before you get wired.

PROS
- Straight teeth make a big difference in your appearance.
- Braces can solve bite problems.
- Straighter teeth are also easier to keep clean and maintain. Crooked or crowded teeth can be a risk factor for PD!

CONS
- Braces can be uncomfortable, socially awkward, and expensive.

BRIGHTER BITERS?
A WHITE SMILE MAKES YOU
(SEEM) SMARTER

Having a beautiful smile can make you seem smarter. Comparison studies between people before and after having their teeth straightened and whitened showed that those with the perfect pearly whites were rated as being more successful, friendly, sensitive, interesting, and intelligent than they were before they had cosmetic dentistry.

Loving Your Looks

Paying attention to, appreciating, and enhancing your skin, hair, and smile over time doesn't mean you're vain. This is all part of creating healthy habits that lay the foundation for lifetime health. By learning to know your body as it matures and seeing how your beauty is changing (not diminishing, but transforming!) over time, you'll learn to take better care of yourself. You'll also become familiar with your body, learn what's natural as it goes through new phases, and become alert to changes that may need a doctor's attention. Making your body (and skin, hair, and teeth) beautiful isn't about searching for a fountain of youth. It's about being healthy, and loving yourself, for your whole life.

4 Happiness Habits

Beating Stress, Depression, and Anxiety

My friend Beth, forty-nine, manages her own conference- and events-planning business and travels all over the country, while *also* managing her husband and two teenagers. It's a busy, demanding, and definitely stressful life. "My life doesn't look like I'm in a commercial for bath salts," she jokes. "But it's an incredible ride."

Beth is like many of my patients in their late thirties, forties, and early fifties. At midlife, their lives are jam-packed with work, family, friends, and other constant demands. Their cell phones are never off; their bosses text them at 10 p.m. The stress is nonstop. (Sound familiar?) And yet they're healthy, strong, and vibrant.

What's going on here? Isn't stress supposed to be bad for you?

The answer is yes . . . and no. Research shows there's good stress and bad stress.

We now know that bad stress—ongoing worries with no end in sight about things that you don't control—is a leading cause of serious chronic illnesses, linked to diabetes, heart disease, and depression. But we also know that some stress, especially short-term stress about events you can control, can actually be good for you. The secret is in knowing which is which, developing strategies for dealing with both kinds, and understanding what it takes for you to stay emotionally healthy.

Fortunately, a growing body of research shows that we can cultivate lifetime habits that help us recognize and deal with stress and negative emotions, helping us live healthier, happier lives. In this chapter, I'll help you understand the latest research on stress and give you a plan to develop lifetime habits to make sure you control your stress—instead of the other way around!

Good and Bad Stress

All stress is not created equal. Certain kinds of stress can actually be good for you, motivating you to do your best, to prepare for challenges, to make strategic decisions about where to spend your time and effort. Many people thrive under pressure. I admit it: I'm one of them. I'm at my best when I'm racing to meet a deadline for a health story while juggling my kids' hockey games, caring for my patients, and squeezing in my almost-daily workouts. But I'm not alone. Lots of writers can't write a word until their deadlines approach. Most professional athletes respond to the stress of competition by delivering their best performances.

This kind of stress can actually be good for you, encouraging you to do your best in every area of your life. Like all stress, good stress triggers the release of chemicals in your body—epinephrine, norepinephrine, adrenaline, and cortisol, a hormone that helps your body retrieve energy from your liver by converting glycogen to glucose. Stress can make us feel surges of energy and give us more focus.

But bad stress, often over events you don't control, can hurt your body over the long haul. Normally, adrenaline and cortisol are your body's friends (especially if you're, say, running away from a man-eating tiger). But if the stress continues for weeks, months, or years, the high levels of cortisol wreak havoc on your body. Cortisol can damage blood vessels, impair your metabolism, affect your overall hormonal balance, delay or impair healing and normal cell growth, and weaken your immune system. With prolonged or chronic stress, a generalized inflammation can set in throughout your body and lead to potentially significant physical problems. No wonder we call this chronic, uncontrolled pressure bad stress.

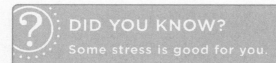

DID YOU KNOW?
Some stress is good for you.

Good stress . . .
- can motivate and energize you.
- is short-term, like a deadline or a crunch period.
- gives you control over the outcome (if you work hard, you can accomplish the goal).
- comes from solvable, short-term problems (like finishing a project at work or cleaning out your basement).

Bad stress . . .
- feels like you have constant nagging problems you can't escape (like a bad boss or deep credit card debt).
- is long-term, day in and day out.
- often surrounds major life transitions, such as moving, divorce, and loss of a loved one; these and long-term financial problems are examples of events that can cause detrimental stress.
- can lead to serious health problems, including heart disease.

CLOCKSTOPPING SECRET: STRESS AGES YOUR BODY

Research has linked stress to a wide variety of physical ills that can age you prematurely, including:

- Diabetes
- Heart disease
- Depression or anxiety
- Migraines or tension headaches
- Gastrointestinal problems (IBS or reflux/heartburn/GERD)
- Asthma
- Increased risk for premature death

TURNING BAD STRESS INTO GOOD

Fortunately, as the medical profession has become more aware of the potentially lethal effects of stress, more and more research has gone into finding ways to control our responses to anxiety, as well as mood problems in general. Today, a wealth of information exists on how to create healthy habits to reduce the effects of stress. We now know that a specific set of habits can help you manage your response to pressure so that it doesn't cause physical or emotional damage. When stress does reach an unmanageable level where you need professional help to regain your balance, these same techniques can work together with therapy and medication to help you feel better faster.

When I talk with my patients about stress, I apply the same philosophy I do with beauty. You need to use every tool in your arsenal to feel your best, emotionally as well as physically. For many people, most of the time that means developing great lifetime habits. But for other patients, that means calling on the best medical and emotional techniques available, from talk therapy with a social worker or psychologist to antidepressant or antianxiety medication to get through difficult periods. While some of my patients resist the idea of professional help or medication to manage their stress or emotions, I tell them that they deserve to feel better, and that emotional health is as important as physical health. If they had high blood pressure, they'd treat that, wouldn't they? Stress, anxiety, and mood disorders are the same. There should be no stigma for seeking help and using every weapon in your arsenal to protect your mental and emotional health.

This chapter will help you develop healthy lifetime stress habits, but also will help you understand when you may need to seek professional help. Either way, the goal is to feel your best emotionally as well as physically, so you can enjoy your beautiful body and beautiful life.

CLOCKSTOPPING SECRET: THE POWER OF SELF-TALK

Here's a secret I use to turn bad stress into good stress. It may sound ridiculously simple, but research shows it works.

When you're under pressure, you may send yourself a lot of bad messages ("This dinner party was a terrible idea. The house is a mess. The food's not turning out well enough. Why don't I plan better?"). It turns out you can often fight all this mental scolding with a flood of positive self-talk. I know it sounds simplistic, but it takes some work and commitment.

If, say, I'm attempting to cook a big dinner for friends and family (and, trust me, I'm the farthest thing from a gourmet chef), I try to shift my focus to my real priorities and goals. I tell myself, "My table doesn't have to look like the Food Channel. What matters isn't a perfect meal. What's important to me here is that I'm welcoming friends and creating community. The dinner doesn't have to be perfect; it just has to be fun." That helps me let go of all the little things that will never be perfect anyway, no matter how much I do. I'm able to enjoy the dinner, have fun with my friends, and simply be happy. And there's no better clockstopper than happiness!

DON'T STRESS OVER STRESS

Reducing stress doesn't mean you have to quit your job. Here's the truth behind three pervasive myths about women and stress.

Myth: Life would be less stressful if you just quit your job.

Truth: Working doesn't stress women out; bad jobs do.

One study shows that working women don't have more heart disease (often linked to stress) than women who stayed home . . . but that women with boring, clerical jobs, or with difficult bosses, do have more heart disease.[1]

Myth: Taking that promotion would stress you out.

Truth: High-power jobs don't necessarily bring bad stress.

A study of twenty-eight thousand people working in the British Civil Service shows that people with low-status jobs, with little control over their work, had much more negative stress than people in higher-status jobs. Even though high-ranking jobs were stressful, workers had more control over their work—and were less likely to die from heart disease.

. . . .

Myth: Type A people have more heart attacks.

Truth: Type A's don't have more stress-related illnesses.

Personally, I was relieved to hear this one. I consider myself a classic type A, as defined by cardiologist Meyer Friedman and his colleague Ray Rosenman in the 1950s as overachieving multitaskers who push themselves hard, meet deadlines, and hate delays. Friedman and Rosenman claimed that type A's were more likely to have negative stress and heart attacks than type B's. But lots of research since then has questioned that assumption (for one thing, they only studied men; for another, there was only a very small difference in heart disease between the two types).

What really matters, more than the type of work you do or the type of personality you have, is how you *recognize, prepare for,* and *respond to* the inevitable stresses that come with a fulfilling, rewarding, fully packed life.

The Body Beautiful Prescription: Stress Relief

Recent research shows that there's a lot you can do to reduce the impact of stress on your life. These habits aren't overnight fixes. They take time and commitment, but the payoff is a happier, healthier life.

WEEK 1: START A DAILY JOURNAL

Having an outlet for your feelings can be hugely helpful to your health, even if you only express them to yourself in the form of writing in a private journal. Developing a lifetime habit of journaling, even if it's just ten minutes every night, can improve your health, reduce your stress, and even help you sleep better.

Numerous studies show that writing—especially about traumatic events—can improve your health.[2] It can also help you perform better under pressure: In one recent experiment, students who wrote about their anxieties on a math test for ten minutes before a test did much better than those who didn't.[3]

This week, your task is to start a journal and write at least one page about what happened to you today. You'll keep this up for the next five weeks and, hopefully, build a lifetime habit.

At the end of each week, read over what you've written, looking for recurring themes, particular events that trigger stress or a bad mood, and generally becoming more aware of factors that make you happy, calm, worried, angry, or tense.

WEEK 2: DEEP BREATHING, TEN MINUTES A DAY

As I mentioned in the beauty chapter, I'm a longtime fan of the Ayurvedic approach to health. Its emphasis on deep breathing to restore balance and wellness falls right in line with a growing body of research showing that deep breathing and meditation are highly effective stress busters. One method in particular can be very helpful: mindfulness meditation, where you focus on the real world around you right now, not the worries in your mind or the constant stream of planning, remembering, ruminating, and imaginary conversations that fill our minds most of the time. Focusing on what your body and senses are experiencing in the present moment, including your breathing, body sensations, and sounds, has been shown by numerous studies to reduce stress, improve mood, and help people react with more equanimity to stressful events.[4]

The good news is that mindful meditation costs nothing and that even just ten minutes a day can make a difference. For a great primer on the benefits and techniques of mindful meditation, as well as free guided meditations, visit the UCLA Mindful Awareness Research Center at marc.ucla.edu.

But you don't have to do a lot of research to start reaping the benefits of mindful meditation practice. Your task for this week is to practice a simple breathing technique, called Ayurvedic breathing, for ten minutes every day. This can be done any time, anywhere. Close your eyes, and gently close one nostril with your middle finger. Breathe in deeply as slowly as possible through the open nostril. At the end of your inhale, release the nostril, close the opposite one with your thumb, and exhale as slowly as possible through the other nostril (the one you had initially covered). Continue for ten minutes, focusing on the feeling of each breath rather than on outside thoughts and worries. If your mind wanders, gently bring it back to think about how each breath feels in your nose, lungs, and body.

In the Ayurvedic tradition, this kind of breathing is thought to unify the right and left sides of your brain and to help bring heart rate, respiratory rate, and blood pressure down. This or any form of meditation can get your mind, body, and spirit in sync and ease your response to stress.

WEEK 3: SCHEDULE A CALL WITH A FRIEND

Research shows that friends and social support are invaluable when fighting stress. One major study showed that when women are stressed, a flood of brain chemicals leads them to "tend and befriend" other women, which releases oxytocin, a chemical that has a calming effect.[5] In lab experiments, isolated animals show more signs of stress and don't live as long as those who live with other animals. Long-term studies show that people with more friends live longer.

So even though calling a friend may seem like the last thing you have time for during stressful periods, your task for this week is to schedule a time to talk with a friend. Put it on your calendar to call, or make a coffee date. It only has to be ten to fifteen minutes—but you'll find making a habit of regular talks with friends lowers your stress and contributes to your lifetime health and well-being.

WEEK 4: MUSIC, ART, DANCING, OR OTHER FUN

By week 4, you're writing in a journal for a few minutes every night, breathing deeply for ten minutes in the morning, and calling a friend once a week. All told, these changes take just a few minutes a day. This week's assignment requires a little more time, but it's well worth it. Think of something creative you've always wanted to do—learn to ballroom dance, play the guitar, sing with a choir, learn French cooking. Find a class or make a date with a friend to try it. Ultimately, I want you to commit to one of these extracurricular activities for a five-week period—and to keep trying out new activities until you find one, just one, that you like and want to stick with. Having some creative outlet that takes your mind completely off your work and your life is one of the healthiest habits you can develop, especially if you're also meditating. One study of 111 women with cancer who combined meditation with art tasks, from self-portraits to clay sculpting, had less stress, less pain, better sleep, and fewer physical complaints than women who did not do the mindful meditation and art program.[6]

You don't have to become Picasso, Yo-Yo Ma, or Mario Batali to reap the stress relief benefits of creativity. All you need to do this week is try a new creative pursuit and stick with it for a few weeks, long enough to see if you enjoy it. If you're not captivated, move on to another new creative activity until you find something completely removed from your daily life to stick with.

WEEK 5: ALTRUISM THERAPY

Pouring your attention into helping others is another good way of treating yourself emotionally. Research shows that when a stressed person focuses on other people, the result is an almost immediate sense of gratification, which over time can reduce stress. In one study of patients with chronic diseases, those patients who served as mentors and confidants to other people with their disease showed more improvement in depression, confidence, and self-esteem than those who did not help their peers.

Your task this week is to spend fifteen to thirty minutes helping someone else. This could be a volunteer project, like reading to kids or visiting the elderly, or simply helping your neighbor with yard work. Make it a practice to do something selfless at least once a week, and you'll find your stress levels drop over time.

AFTER FIVE WEEKS

Remember, the five-week program is meant to encourage you to build a series of healthy habits that you'll maintain over time. With this program, it's particularly important to do another five-week cycle where you practice all five of the new habits I recommend here. That's because some of these habits, like creative pursuits and altruism, work over a long period of time, so you want to be sure to give them a good long chance. My hope is that with time, some or all of these will become a permanent part of your life.

COMFORT FOODS

Okay, so we all know we're not supposed to eat or drink our cares away. But . . . what if it's healthy food? Some healthy foods can be terrific stress busters. While it's important to realize that no food or drink can *cure* stress or a true mood disorder, you may be able to reduce the effects of stress with a trip to your grocery store.

Whole-grain oatmeal: Packed with the healthy type of complex carbohydrates, this may work as a mood stabilizer by boosting the feel-good brain chemical serotonin.

Low-fat milk: The calcium found in milk is helpful in reducing muscle spasms and can ease anxiety and boost mood. (Drink it warm for a more relaxing effect.)

Sushi: This packs a great combo of protein and B-complex vitamins in the fish and the serotonin-boosting carbohydrates and fiber found in the rice. Salmon in particular can help to balance cortisol levels.

Avocados: These are filled with potassium, which can help lower blood pressure, and also contain the healthy type of monounsaturated fat. Half of an avocado has more potassium than a medium-sized banana.

Oranges: The vitamin C in this citrus fruit helps keep cortisol in check.

Nuts: High in B vitamins, which are used in the body's stress response, and also the antioxidant vitamin E, nuts are a great source of protein.

Spinach: Rich in magnesium, spinach can help reduce headaches caused by stress and combat the fatigue that can accompany stress.

GENDER STRESS: HOW WOMEN AND MEN DIFFER

Research done at the University of Pennsylvania Perelman School of Medicine has shown that there are actual differences in the brain activity of men and women under stressful conditions.[7] In women confronted with short-term stress, the area of the brain that is primarily associated with emotional responses (called the limbic system) becomes highly activated. In stressed-out men, however, the frontal regions of the cerebral cortex tend to become active. These regions control executive functions such as decision making, moderating complex social behavior, and coordinating thoughts with actions. This may explain the gender generalization that many women respond to stress emotionally while men tend to respond more systematically. (But let's not forget this is a generalization! Lots of men respond emotionally to stress, whether they show it or not, and plenty of women show stone-cold logic under duress.)

Unfortunately, for women, stress may be complicated by the ebb and flow of our hormones, especially as we age. The brain contains receptors for the powerful female hormone estrogen (more accurately referred to as estradiol, but we'll use the more familiar term). Any fluctuation in hormone levels can affect mood (as we know from the existence of PMS). Our moods and response to stress, then, may feel more extreme as we age, approach menopause, and experience changes in estrogen levels. Fortunately, simply realizing that your response to stress may have a chemical component may help you put things into perspective: It may make your symptoms seem less random, easier to control, and, perhaps, easier for professionals to help manage.

Seeking Help

No matter how good your stress management habits are, life will throw you curveballs—death, divorce, illness, or even hormonal and chemical changes in your body can plunge you into depression or anxiety that you just can't shake. A period of prolonged stress may exacerbate old or underlying psychological disorders. Anxiety or depression can get worse; so can eating disorders, obsessive-compulsive behaviors, substance abuse problems, or compulsive or addictive habits like gambling, binge eating, or spending.

If your stress seems to have consumed you, if your moods seem to be stretching out into longer and longer low points, or if your stress or anxiety is interfering with your daily responsibilities, you may need to see a therapist or other mental health professional. There are emotional and mood disorders that no amount of good intentions and healthy habits can shake: You *cannot* think your way out of clinical depression. Asking for help is the first step in getting better. The time has long since passed when you need to feel embarrassed about asking for help with moods, behavior, or mental imbalances. After all, if you had the flu, you'd go to the doctor, right?

Options for treatment of stress, anxiety, depression, and mood disorders depend on the type of problem you are experiencing and the type of mental health professional who makes you feel comfortable. A licensed social worker, psychotherapist, psychologist (a Ph.D.), or a psychiatrist (an M.D.) can all be helpful in treating stress and mood disorders, ranging from mild to extreme issues. Usually, rather than telling you what to do, these professionals will help *you* discover your own way of coping. If medication is necessary, either in the form of a mood stabilizer, sleep aid, or antianxiety medication, a doctor would prescribe it and monitor you to see if you improve or suffer side effects.

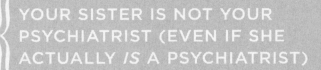

YOUR SISTER IS NOT YOUR PSYCHIATRIST (EVEN IF SHE ACTUALLY *IS* A PSYCHIATRIST)

Many people mistakenly believe that simply talking about their problems with friends or family can relieve their emotional distress. While this may help, it's very important to know that your friends and family can never be completely objective. That's why I feel it's very important to find a therapist—a psychologist, psychiatrist, or social worker—who does not know you or your cast of characters personally. You'll be able to say things or admit things you'd never confide in the people closest to you. And the best part is, this person is there only for *you*. What a luxury!

ASSESS YOUR STRESS

When I talk with my patients, I always ask them about their stress, anxiety, and depression levels. I believe in treating the whole patient, and that includes understanding whether emotional disorders or unmanageable stress may be undermining their physical or emotional health. I usually ask a series of questions, similar to those I've listed in the quiz below, to get a sense of their emotional health. I've included these questions and an explanation about how I think about the answers to give you rough guidelines on how to determine how much stress you're under, and whether or not you may benefit from professional help. This is my own assessment, and certainly not the final word on whether you should seek counseling or not. If you score well, but still have a sense that you'd benefit from talking to a professional, I strongly urge you to try it. If you have any doubts, talk to your doctor.

1. Do you have any areas in your life that are providing stress?
   ☐ Yes ☐ No

2. Do you have stress in your family/home life? ☐ Yes ☐ No

3. Do you have stress in your work/career? ☐ Yes ☐ No

4. Do you have stress in your physical condition/health?
   ☐ Yes ☐ No

5. Do you have stress in your social life (with friends/relationships)?
   ☐ Yes ☐ No

6. Have there been any major changes lately or are any anticipated?
   ☐ Yes ☐ No

7. Are you getting married or divorced? ☐ Yes ☐ No

8. Are you having a baby? ☐ Yes ☐ No

9. Is someone you care about ill or dying? ☐ Yes ☐ No

10. Are you getting a promotion or demotion at work?
    ☐ Yes ☐ No

11. Are you moving? ☐ Yes ☐ No

12. Are you able to perform your basic daily activities without too
    much disruption caused by emotional distress? This means you
    are able to get up, shower, feed yourself and/or your family, go to
    work, and address your responsibilities. ☐ Yes ☐ No

13. Have you noticed any changes in the way you feel, eat, or sleep?
    ☐ Yes ☐ No

14. Have you been sleeping more or less? ☐ Yes ☐ No

15. Have you been eating more or less? ☐ Yes ☐ No

16. Have you engaged in any recent behaviors that you would
    describe as risky (ranging from spending sprees to contacting old
    lovers when you're still in a committed relationship to drug use)?
    ☐ Yes ☐ No

17. Are you drinking more alcohol than usual or more than twice a
    day? ☐ Yes ☐ No

18. Are you taking prescription medication for relaxation or anxiety
    to help you get through the day? ☐ Yes ☐ No

Scoring

If you answered *yes* to:

- **0–3 questions:** Congratulations, guru! You're an oasis of inner
  peace, with little or no stress.
- **4–5 questions:** Like most of us, you have a manageable amount of
  stress—and remember, some stress is good!
- **6–7 questions:** Your life seems a little more stressful than average,
  but you seem to be coping. You might consider therapy or stress-
  reduction techniques like meditation or yoga.
- **8–10 questions:** Severe stress alert. You may be overloaded with
  more stressful events than you can handle. It's a good idea to seek
  help from multiple sources. Increase stress-relieving activities,

like yoga and spending time with friends. Meanwhile, talk to your doctor, and ask friends for referrals to therapists or counselors. If your employer offers an Employee Assistance Program (EAP), call the confidential number, explain that you're looking for help coping with stress and anxiety, and ask for a referral. Your insurance company may also have stress management or mental health resources.

11-18 questions: Your stress level is extreme. You need professional help. Call your doctor and pursue the other ideas listed above right away. There is no shame or stigma in knowing when you need help and finding the resources that can make you feel better. You owe it to yourself and your loved ones to find help.

Be Unconflicted

My own life is pretty busy and, yes, stressful: I have two active kids. My husband and I both have demanding jobs. I'm responsible for my patients' health. I share important health information with viewers on national television. I write books and articles, and make personal appearances in support of various charities. I have lots of friends and family to keep up with.

People ask me all the time how I balance all this.

My answer is just two words: Be unconflicted. The thing that gets me through is a rock-solid understanding of my priorities. My family comes first. Period. Then, my patients and the viewers with whom I share important medical information. Knowing that helps me stay committed to taking care of myself and reducing stress. Putting someone or something first that doesn't or can't reciprocate can often lead to more stress, hurt, and disappointment, so choose wisely. I know if I falter physically or emotionally, everything and everyone depending on me may fall down, too, like a row of dominoes. That sounds like a lot of pressure, I know—but actually, it helps me remember how important it is to manage my stress. So I make sure I take care of myself. I wouldn't be a good mom, wife, or doctor if I were unhealthy, moody, or distracted.

This is why I believe that, for women especially, being unconflicted about your priorities is a vital step toward restoring your inner and outer balance in times of stress. Remember what matters to you and, when you're stressed or struggling, get back on track to serving those people or roles. Taking care of yourself first and foremost isn't selfish. It's actually the opposite! It allows you to be fully present in every situation. By being 100 percent in the moment, you will be more able to push through stressful times or experiences.

You can't be your best self or do your best work if you're distracted, stressed, or conflicted, so understand what really matters to you. Deal with the things that you *can* control, and don't worry about the things you can't. If this means saying no, or doing less, there's no shame in that. One of my patients whose husband was battling an aggressive form of cancer was so focused on taking care of him and her children that she neglected herself. While I couldn't do anything to help his cancer, I did send her a gift certificate for a massage, because I knew she would never get one for herself. Sometimes taking a moment to recharge your body and spirit is all that's needed to help address even chronic long-term stress.

5

The Body Beautiful Prescription for Better Sex

Many of my married patients in their thirties and forties tell me they only have sex when they're on vacation. I tell them to take more vacations! Research shows that a happy sex life is linked to overall good health. Not only can it help you feel younger and healthier, it can make you look younger, too!

But sex, however powerful, is different in our thirties and forties than it might have been in our twenties. The good news is, sex can actually be *better* as you age, because you really know who you are and what you want. On the other hand, most women find themselves much busier and more stressed in their thirties and forties. We have less time for ourselves, and less time and energy for sex. Often, we're in a committed relationship, so the novelty and excitement may have given way to work, family, and routine. This explains the vacation sex phenomenon: When you're away, you're relaxed, not distracted by kids or work or the dishes, and have time to appreciate each other. If you can learn to create the same mental space at home, you'll be well on your way to better sex *and* better health!

Most of my patients are surprised to hear that sex doesn't have to diminish over time, and that even after a long dry spell, there are specific things you can do to turn things around. Surprisingly, sex is a lot like eating and exercise; it's all about developing good habits.

My patients aren't usually accustomed to thinking about sex as something to work on. After all, that doesn't sound romantic or spontaneous. But the fact is, when life gets busy, sex rarely happens as effortlessly as it once did. As you age, sex requires attention, care, and above all, good physical, mental, and emotional health.

Taking time to think about your sex life, improve it, and nurture it are key processes in keeping your body beautiful inside and out. Building a beautiful sex life is not selfish. You don't have to be embarrassed. And you can enjoy satisfying results very soon. You deserve it. And trust me—it's worth the effort!

CLOCKSTOPPING SECRET: MORE SEX MAKES YOU LOOK YOUNGER

One study by researchers in Scotland asked observers to guess the ages of more than thirty-five hundred people. The people who had the most sex also looked much younger than their real ages—four to seven years younger!

Why? One theory is that sex boosts the production of human growth hormone, which in turn improves muscle tone and makes you look younger and more fit. Other studies show that more sex is associated with greater happiness, a stronger immune system, and longer life.

Sexing It Up

During any routine exam, I ask my patients how their sex lives are going. Given that an estimated 43–90 percent of women have sexual worries at some point in their lives, ranging from lack of desire to inability to achieve orgasm, it's not surprising that my patients almost always seem relieved to talk about sex. They're even more relieved when they find out that there are specific things they can do to improve their desire for, and enjoyment of, sex. I created a plan for my patients to help them improve their sexual habits and give them the sex lives they want. Usually, we start with this quiz. Try it yourself to see where you stand.

Quiz: How's Your Sex Life?

Over the past month:

1. How many times did you have sex?

(a) Never   (b) Once or twice all month   (c) Once a week or more

2. Have you experienced any vaginal dryness?

(a) Always   (b) Occasionally   (c) Never

3. Have you had any pain during intercourse?

(a) Frequently   (b) Occasionally   (c) Never

4. How would you describe your desire for sex?

(a) Low   (b) Moderate   (c) High

5. Are you satisfied with your sex life?

(a) No   (b) It's okay   (c) Yes, it's great!

6. Are you satisfied with your ability to become aroused?
(a) No, it's a problem   (b) Somewhat satisfied   (c) Yes

7. Are you satisfied with your ability to have/the frequency of an orgasm?
(a) No   (b) Somewhat satisfied   (c) Yes

8. Even if you have low desire, once you start having sex, are you able to enjoy it?
(a) Not at all satisfied   (b) Not really—I would rather be doing something else   (c) Yes

Give yourself one point for each A, two points for each B, and three points for each C. Add up your points and look at the grading system below.

22–24: Grade: A. Whatever you're doing, patent it!

20–22: Grade: B. You're probably the envy of most of your friends. Keep it going!

18–20: Grade: C. Not bad, but there's definitely room for improvement.

16–18: Grade: D. Your sex life could use some TLC.

Less than 16: Grade: F: Your sex life needs CPR. Read on for advice on resuscitating your sex life.

LOW LIBIDO OR HIGH STRESS?

Many of my patients in their thirties and forties tell me they just don't feel much desire for their partner. Is something medically wrong with them?

There *is* an official, clinical condition describing low libido: hypoactive sexual desire disorder. You may be suffering from it if you have a persistent or recurrent lack of sexual desire causing "significant distress or interpersonal difficulty."[1] What's interesting is the "distress or difficulty" part. If your partner has the same pattern of desire, you may not really have a problem—even if you only have sex a few times a year!

On the other hand, if your low levels of desire are causing tension with your partner, or if you're just worried and disappointed with the sex life you have, you owe it to yourself and your relationship to consider the causes behind your low libido. All kinds of things can cause a drop in your sex drive, from common medications (like birth control pills or antidepressants—ironically, low libido might make you more depressed) to situations (like relationship problems or chronic illnesses). If you think you have a libido problem, speaking to a doctor or a sex therapist can be very helpful in isolating and defining the problem and correcting the situation.

CLOCKSTOPPING SECRET: SEX IS GOOD FOR YOUR BODY[2]

Just a few more ways that sex keeps your body young and healthy:

Boosts Your Immune System. Research shows that people who have sex once or twice a week have higher levels of immunoglobulin A in their blood, which results in better immune protection.

Promotes Good Circulation. Frequent orgasms stimulate the release of the precursor hormone DHEA, which helps circulation and promotes healthy levels of estrogen and testosterone.

Burns Calories. At approximately 5 calories per minute (depending on your weight), one hour of horizontal aerobic activity can burn

more than 300 calories. Even a quickie can burn off a cookie (well, a
small one).

Helps You Live Longer. Studies at Duke University have shown that
women who really enjoyed their sex lives lived seven to eight years
longer than women who were indifferent about sex.

RULE OUT MEDICAL CAUSES

Usually when one of my patients is having a sexual problem, it's caused
by one of three things: a physical or medical issue, including pain; a
lifestyle issue, including young children and hectic schedules, which
can contribute to an inability to get in the mood, sexual boredom, or
both; or last, an unknown cause.

I tackle the physical issues first. I evaluate medications that my
patients take, since many medications, from antidepressants to blood
pressure medications to herbal supplements, can affect libido. Ask your
doctor if anything you're taking could be contributing to sexual
problems.

Next, a good physical examination will check for anything that could
be causing physical pain or sexual problems. This could range from
pelvic infections to uterine fibroids to vaginal infections to vulvar skin
conditions. Sometimes bacterial cultures, urine cultures, or a pelvic ultrasound may be helpful.

ASSESS YOUR LIFE

If there are no medical reasons for the sexual problem, we look at lifestyle factors. Is there a young baby or toddler waking you up at night—
or even sleeping in your bed? Are you being distracted by your teenager
or worried about your college student? Or are you just so exhausted

when you lie down that the very last thing on your mind is sex? All of these are real and potentially powerful factors that can put your desire on ice. Women are classic multitaskers, but when it comes to sexual desire, we need to have a clear mind in order to have even an inkling of interest in sex. When a woman is busy with work, bills, laundry, errands, kids, and extended family, the last thing on her mind is getting busy in the bedroom. (This explains the vacation sex phenomenon again!)

If you find lifestyle factors are interfering, brainstorm ways you can work around them. Meanwhile, start following the five-week plan to better sex. (Note: My plan assumes that you're in a committed relationship. That's because the majority of my patients in their thirties or forties have long-term partners, and their concerns revolve around protecting and improving the physical aspects of their relationship over the years.)

The Body Beautiful Prescription: Five Weeks to Sexy Habits

WEEK 1: GET OUT YOUR CALENDAR

Fortunately, you don't need to go to Hawaii to improve your sex life. The answer is as close as your day planner. Sex therapists recommend scheduling sex. This might not sound romantic or spontaneous, but it really works.

First, putting it on your calendar compartmentalizes sex. That is, it gives you a clear, defined space and time when you and your partner are not checking your iPhones. Second, scheduling sex can actually increase desire. If you write it down, you'll have it on your mind. The idea will percolate all day, triggering and increasing desire. When you think about sex, you are more likely to want to have sex. So your task during the first week is simply to schedule a date night every week for the next five weeks. If you miss it, be sure to reschedule. Simply committing to sex once a week and planning when you'll have it will start moving your body and mind in the right direction. (Your partner may resist this idea as being unromantic, but ask him to humor you. You can promise he'll enjoy the results!)

WEEK 2: PELVIC REHAB—USE IT OR LOSE IT

So let's assume that you *want* to have sex, but once you start, you find it difficult to become aroused. This is very common among patients who haven't had sex in a while or who've been suffering from low libido. Your pelvis and genitals may literally be out of practice. Like any other muscle group, the muscles, nerves, and glands in your pelvis function at their best when they're used regularly. In other words, the more sex you have, the better it gets. Ironically, the cure for sexual problems may be having sex more often, not less!

I call this positive feedback cycle, where use improves function, pelvic rehab. Before you know it, those muscles are back in shape, the nerves have come out of hibernation, and the glands are back to work, secreting lubricant fluids.

Your sexual rehab program has two steps. Start this week and keep it up for the next four.

Kegels: Kegels are exercises for your pelvic floor. By strengthening these muscles, you tone and "wake up" your pelvic area, which may help you achieve orgasm more readily and prevent low libido. They're simple: Just contract the same muscles you use when you're trying not to pee. Hold the contraction for five seconds, then relax for five seconds. Work up to a ten-second hold and a ten-second break. Your goal is to do three sets of ten kegels every day (or more!).

Eliminate vaginal dryness: Arousal problems often center around vaginal dryness, poor lubrication, or decreased genital sensation. Treatment for dryness is very individual: Different women respond to different solutions. I recommend my patients try one of three cheap-and-easy remedies: saliva (it works!), over-the-counter lubricants such as K-Y or Durex Play Utopia, or all-natural essential oils like Zestra or sunflower oil.

Sometimes vaginal dryness results from low estrogen levels. This is common while breast-feeding and close to menopause. As a remedy, a low-dose, bioidentical estrogen cream can be applied vaginally with minimal to no absorption into your bloodstream. The added estrogen can really rejuvenate the vagina. If dryness is a persistent problem, talk to your doctor about estrogen cream.

WEEK 3: FANTASIZE

Your prescription this week: Fantasize for ten minutes a day. That may sound silly, but the idea is sound. When you focus your mind on sex, your body will follow. For this to work, you need to know what excites you. Some of my patients find racy novels get them all steamed up. Others like movies or pictures (there's a *reason* that pornography is the world's most profitable industry). Give yourself permission to imagine scenes and setups that excite you. Don't be embarrassed: Nobody ever has to know (although I highly recommend you try sharing some of your fantasies with your partner . . . the results may astonish you). The important thing is the physical process that fantasizing launches in your body, warming you up and making you more physically prepared for arousal and orgasm. The key is to stop thinking about arousal as something that happens ten minutes before you have sex, and to think about it as a process that may start hours or even days before your actual sex date (which should be on your calendar by now!).

WEEK 4: GOOD VIBRATIONS

This week your assignment is to try vibrator therapy. I'm not kidding! Using a vibrator can help rehab the nerves in the vagina and clitoris. I often recommend this to my patients who have had cancer and been treated with pelvic radiation, which can damage nerve fibers. Because a vibrator can produce high-frequency, precise stimulation for unlimited amounts of time and is under your control, it can be a very effective way to resuscitate the nerves and tissue in the genital region. Vibrators can be particularly helpful for women who have painful intercourse, since the woman can control penetration, speed, and pressure. So don't be hesitant to get yourself a vibrator. You can start by using it yourself, and then use it with your partner when and if you'd like.

Don't have the first clue about where to get one? A website called Babeland (www.babeland.com) is reputable, respectable, not sleazy, and lets you buy products in the privacy of your own home. It also provides customer reviews of various models.

Of course, you may not need or want a vibrator to help you reach your own orgasm. Masturbation is a natural, normal practice and extremely helpful in teaching you how your body responds to physical stimulation. After all, how will you know what you want from your partner if you can't do it yourself? By using your hands or a vibrator, you can explore your own body and what feels good. When you start to enjoy pleasure on your own, you will be better able to enjoy sex.

The important principle here is that the more sensual you are on your own, the more sensual you'll be with your partner.

WEEK 5: EXPERIMENT

This week, use your imagination and try something new. Just one rule: Don't do anything that would be emotionally or physically hurtful to you or your partner. That leaves a lot of latitude. You don't have to swing from a chandelier or think you have to re-create the sex life you see in a movie or on TV. For some people, experimenting might be having sex with the lights on, or in the kitchen. Here are some ideas:

- Sexy lingerie
- Costumes
- Use a silk tie as a blindfold
- Try a striptease or naked dance for/with your partner
- Try a new position or one you haven't done in a while
- Ask for something: Your experiment could be as simple as asking your partner to do something you like.

For more ideas, visit www.drlauraberman.com. Laura Berman is a sex therapist at Northwestern University. She has lots of ideas (including sex toy suggestions) on her website.

 TALKING IS SEXY

Good communication between you and your partner is an essential part of a healthy and fulfilling sex life. This requires a certain level of comfort with the expression of your desires and fantasies. I know this can be hard if you and your partner aren't used to talking, or if you've become less connected in the crazy business of work and family. You might broach the subject playfully, saying, "You know, I read this book that says sex makes you healthier . . . and says we should schedule it once a week.

Wanna try?" You might be watching TV with a steamy scene and happen to mention that you'd like to try something like that. Or just have a glass of wine and say how much you liked something you did together recently, or that there's something you'd like to try. There are lots of ways to open the conversation. The key is to become comfortable talking about what you want and to acknowledge to each other that great sex is an important part of life, and something you both want to share for a long time. Not only can these conversations bring a relationship closer together, but they can also have a positive impact on your self-esteem. It shows your partner, and yourself, that you are a woman who knows what she wants and is not afraid or ashamed to ask for it. That sense of confidence can be a *big* turn-on to you both.

Where's the Little Pink Pill for Women?

What if you've exhausted all of the aforementioned do-it-yourself remedies for your sexual problem and you're still not swinging from a trapeze in the bedroom? Why isn't there a simple pill you can pop? It just doesn't seem fair that when men suffer sexual problems, all they need to do is see their doctor for a quick and easy prescription for an erectile dysfunction medication like Viagra and be happily on their way. (Unless, of course, they have one of those four-hour erections as a side effect. Then they'd be *unhappily* on their way—to the emergency room!) Why doesn't the same treatment exist for women? Where's *our* little pink pill?

Unfortunately, it's not that simple. For women, sexual dysfunction is a much more complex problem than it is for men. It doesn't help that less scientific research has been done on women's sexual function than men's. We understand erections much better than we understand female arousal and orgasm. For men, when there's an issue downstairs, it's usually a "plumbing" problem. Improve blood flow to the penis and most men are good to go. For women, sexual problems can originate in the brain (for desire) or the pelvis (for nerve transmission or lubrication), and are therefore much more complicated to treat. (Also, it helps to remember that it's not really that simple for men, either. Drugs like Viagra don't do anything to give a man desire or increase libido. If a man doesn't want sex, being able to have a long, hard erection isn't going to change that. Viagra doesn't solve everything.)

In some ways, Viagra may be complicating women's sexual concerns. After all, if a man takes a pill that unleashes his performance in the bedroom, what happens to his partner, especially if she's struggling with her own sexual difficulties? If she doesn't want to have sex, and suddenly he's able to make love like a twenty-year-old again, couldn't that stack the deck against them, or move her toward *more* sexual anxieties and problems? It's a complicated and interesting dilemma.

One thing's for sure: Despite major financial motivation for big pharmaceutical companies to discover a drug that works for women, no one's yet discovered a miracle pill, although several drugs have been studied in women for treating low libido or problems with achieving orgasm. Studies have shown varying results and none has been FDA approved.

Viagra itself, as well as similar drugs, is now used off-label (that is, in a way not approved by the FDA) by women, but the results are inconsistent. For men, these drugs work by increasing blood flow to the genitals. They do the same for women. Several studies have shown that Viagra, when given to women who have trouble becoming aroused, was effective in 40–80 percent of them. One study looked at women who suffered low libido after taking depression medication. Among them, 72 percent who took Viagra said their sexual function improved. Among women who took a sugar pill, about 27 percent reported improvement.[3]

But there were several caveats with this particular study, as with others, and the side effects of drugs like Viagra, like headache and flushing, can be significant. Meanwhile, other studies have shown no improvement. For all these reasons, women should not take Viagra without consulting with their doctor.

Antidepressants have also been studied for the treatment of women's sexual dysfunction, with inconclusive results. A drug called Flibanserin, which was ineffective for treating depression, was studied in women with hypoactive sexual desire disorder (low sex drive). When given over a twenty-four-week period in a study funded by the drug manufacturer, those women who took the drug did report an improvement in their sexual desire and sexual satisfaction compared with those not taking the drug. However, 15 percent of women taking the drug experienced *very* serious side effects, including depression and even loss of consciousness! Obviously, the drug was not approved.

There *is* one treatment that seems to be showing some promise in treating female sexual dysfunction: the supplement DHEA. DHEA is a precursor to the hormones estrogen and testosterone and is the most abundant circulating steroid in humans. In a clinical trial, postmenopausal women were given low doses of vaginal DHEA (where the pill was inserted in the vagina and absorbed vaginally, not orally) for twelve weeks. Compared with women given a placebo, women who used DHEA had improvement in all aspects of their sexual function: desire, arousal, orgasm, and vaginal dryness/pain. They did not experience any increase in levels of testosterone, estrogen, or DHEA above the normal range.

Even though this study was done in women whose average age was fifty-eight, it's possible that DHEA may be helpful for younger women as well, and more research is being done. Unfortunately, it can be difficult to find low doses of DHEA, as most supplements intended for oral use are much higher. (The study tested three different low dosages: 3.5 mg, 6 mg, and 12 mg.) Since higher doses of DHEA can affect hormone levels, be sure to discuss any and all supplements you take with your doctor.[4]

Last, probably the most requested treatment for female sexual dysfunction (especially low libido) is testosterone. Many women, and men, think that simply supplying more of this hormone will solve all sexual problems. Though not FDA approved for treating low libido, testosterone given via the skin (through a transdermal patch) has been shown to be effective in improving sexual desire when used short-term (for less than six months). Since the risks of testosterone can be significant (like growing hair in various places, deepening of the voice, acne, increased cholesterol, and possibly a risk of breast cancer), you should carefully weigh the possible benefits versus these risks with your doctor.

Better Sex for a Better Life

Whether you and your partner make love once a day, once a week, or once a month, a healthy sex life is a key element in living a beautiful, fulfilling life. Your sex life doesn't have to resemble a porn movie or a racy novel, either. As long as you and your partner are communicating, expressing yourselves, and making each other feel good in your time together, you'll reap the physical and emotional benefits for years to come.

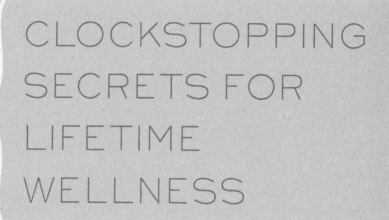

CLOCKSTOPPING
SECRETS FOR
LIFETIME
WELLNESS

Stopping the Clock on Disease

Congratulations! If you've read this far, you know how to create healthy habits for yourself and you have a series of five-week plans to help you focus on specific changes. All of these five-week programs are focused on making the most of your body's own beauty, stopping the clock on aging, and laying a foundation for future health so you stay healthy, vibrant, and strong for the rest of your life.

Part of stopping the clock on your body and staying vibrant and beautiful in every decade is avoiding the most common diseases that affect women as we age. Science now knows a great deal about the causes of major killers, from breast cancer to heart disease. New research is coming out every day about factors that seem to protect us against these diseases, which become more common as we age. As you read the next section, look for boxes explaining the habits you need to develop to help protect yourself against these diseases.

It's important to know that even the best protective habits, like maintaining a healthy weight and an active lifestyle, don't mean you won't get breast cancer, heart disease, or other illnesses. Statistically, these habits reduce your odds, but they're no guarantee. They're a lot like seat belts. Wearing one makes you statistically safer, but it doesn't mean that you won't get hurt in an accident.

It's no coincidence that many of these habits (maintaining a healthy weight, exercising every day, eating healthfully) are the focus of the five-week Body Beautiful prescriptions. These habits all work together, contributing to overall inner and outer beauty, not just in your thirties and forties, but throughout your entire life.

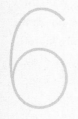

Sexual Health Makeover

Contraception and STIs in Your Thirties and Forties

dmit it: You're thinking about skipping this chapter. Birth control, safe sex—you've got it covered.

But stick around and read on. There's new information here that you need to know. You should review and update your contraceptive needs in your thirties and forties, because new options are on the market. There's also new information on sexually transmitted infections (STIs) that you need to know, even if you're *positive* your partner is monogamous.

Contraceptive Update

In the last few years, your options for birth control have expanded, and they continue to change. The contraception that's right for you depends largely on your age and your family status (single, married, want more kids, or not). In this section, I've listed some of the most common options by the types of patients most likely to need them.

In my practice, most of my patients in their thirties or forties fall into one of four groups: single women who are dating; women with kids who might want more, but not right now; women with no kids, who want them; and those who don't want kids at all or who have enough. Here's what I recommend.

PROFILE 1: SINGLE AND DATING

If you're single, sexually active, and haven't hit menopause, you absolutely must use *two* forms of birth control. You need to use condoms to prevent STIs, and one of the methods I describe below to prevent unwanted pregnancies. Short of abstinence, condoms are the only way to decrease the risk of STIs.

Condoms

Pros: Inexpensive and easy to use. Decrease the risk of sexually transmitted infections. Very popular, even with married couples.

Cons: 17 percent failure rate with typical use. (Yep, 17 percent failure. That means seventeen out of a hundred times, they break, leak, or slip. You may not even know that it happened until you're unexpectedly pregnant or stuck with an STI.)

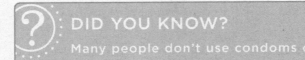

? DID YOU KNOW?
Many people don't use condoms correctly.

Be sure there's space left for semen at the tip, and hold on to the base after sex is finished and until the penis is out of your body.

PROFILE 2: ALREADY HAVE KIDS . . .
AND MIGHT WANT MORE

Recommendation: Low-dose birth control pills or condoms

If you started taking the pill as a teenager, chances are they're a little different now. Some pills today contain just 20 percent of the amount of estrogen that pills in the seventies or eighties contained. That means fewer side effects. Another new trend is the twenty-four-day pill, rather than the older twenty-one-day method. The older method includes a full week of sugar pills, or placebos. Called the pill-free interval, this week off all hormones is when your period comes. But research has shown that women don't need seven days off from active pills. In fact, four days off is enough. (Some forms of the pill now exist where you get your period even less often.) In my practice, I have found that this shorter pill-free interval helps women suffering from PMS or menstrual migraines to avoid those big hormonal triggers. So don't be surprised if you open up a new prescription of pills and find it looks a bit different than it used to. Twenty-four-day pill regimens are now pretty common.

No matter what regimen you're on, the pill is more than 99 percent effective with perfect use—that is, if you never, ever miss a pill and if you always take it at the exact same time every day. But who's perfect? If you miss a pill now and then or don't take it at the same time every day (we call this "typical use"), the pill has an 8 percent failure rate.

Oral Contraceptives

Pros: Reversible. You can stop taking the pill and try to get pregnant right away. Periods are shorter, lighter, and less painful. Protects against ovarian and uterine cancers and ovarian cysts. Clears up acne.

Cons: Increased risk of blood clots. (This risk rises significantly if you smoke and are over thirty-five. If you fall in this group, the pill is *not* recommended.) Can be expensive, up to $70 or more a month. Be sure to ask your doctor for samples, discount prescription cards, or if a cheaper, generic form exists.

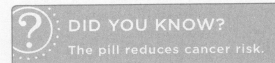

DID YOU KNOW?
The pill reduces cancer risk.

The pill can lower your chances of developing ovarian and uterine cancers. Read chapter 12 for more details.

PROFILE 3: WOMEN WHO WANT KIDS WITHIN A FEW YEARS

Recommendation: NuvaRing, the pill, or condoms

For patients who definitely want to get pregnant in the future, but not right now, a temporary form of birth control is best. Condoms and the pill are good options, but so is the NuvaRing. This is a silicon ring that you insert in your vagina, where it sits for three weeks, releasing low doses of hormones.

NuvaRing

Pros: You don't have to remember to take a pill every day; insert it once, then remove it three weeks later for a week. Can be left in or removed during sex, and if removed can stay out for up to four hours. Bypasses the liver's metabolism, minimizing effects on cholesterol or clotting factors. Offers the same protective factors as the pill.

Cons: Offers the same risk factors as the pill.

PROFILE 4.1: STRAIGHT WOMEN OR LESBIANS WHO DON'T WANT KIDS

Recommendation: Any of the above

For women who have never had children and don't intend to, I still recommend the pill. Sometimes this surprises my lesbian patients, because many lesbians and their doctors automatically assume that if there's no penis involved in sex, contraception is unnecessary. As far as preventing pregnancy goes, that's true. But the pill does much more than reduce the chances of becoming pregnant, including reducing the risk of ovarian and uterine cancers. For women who are either straight or gay who never want children, that protection could be even more important, because never having a full-term pregnancy increases the risk of both kinds of cancer.

Meanwhile, it goes without saying that women who are bisexual—even if they only sleep with a man once in a blue moon—absolutely need birth control if they don't want to become pregnant. Like any other sexually active woman, they should use both condoms (to prevent STIs) and a backup method.

DON'T TAKE THE PILL IF . . .

Some women should never take birth control pills, including:

- smokers over thirty-five years old (btw, you should quit smoking).
- women over thirty-five with a history of classic migraines or migraines with auras.
- women who are obese or who have high blood pressure.
- women of any age with a family history of a clotting disorder.
- women with breast cancer.

PROFILE 4.2: WOMEN WHO WANT PERMANENT CONTRACEPTION

If you're absolutely sure you never want kids (or any *more* kids), we can talk about permanent contraception. Both you, and your husband if you're married, have options.

Before explaining them, I want to say a few things about this choice. This is a personal and individual decision. There is no correct age, no correct number of children to have had . . . but there are some facts you should know. Surgical sterilization via tying the fallopian tubes (called a tubal ligation), blocking the tubes (with the Essure method), or male vasectomy are all considered to be permanent. Although it is technically possible to reverse these procedures, it is not without risks, expense, and possible failure. Usually, when one of my patients discusses surgical sterilization with me, we revisit the topic several times before making the appointment to go ahead with the procedure. In other words, it is not done on a whim. So think carefully and be absolutely sure before you do it.

Women have two options for permanent contraception: tying the tubes (via a number of different methods) or blocking the tubes (via the Essure method).

Tubal Ligation

Tubal ligation is done through a small incision in the belly button. The fallopian tubes are tied and then cut on each side. In a slightly different procedure, one to three half-inch incisions are made in the abdomen under general anesthesia. A laparoscope is inserted and a silicone ring is placed around each fallopian tube, forming a loop or knuckle of a blocked segment of tube.

> Pros: If done right, your chances of getting pregnant are very low: seven to ten in a thousand. (That's right—even permanent contraception can fail sometimes! For this reason, I always tell patients that if you ever miss a period, take a pregnancy test immediately.)
>
> Cons: If a pregnancy *does* occur after getting a tubal ligation, there's a higher chance of a tubal or ectopic pregnancy, which requires immediate treatment.

While tubal ligation is a quick and simple surgical procedure, don't forget that *all* surgery has small but real risks. Other organs in the pelvis, including the intestines, bladder, and blood vessels, may be damaged. And the process is done under general anesthesia, which carries its own risks, including a small risk of death. For these reasons, even though I have performed this operation many, many times, I recommend my patients consider other options first.

Essure

For the past decade, a second method of sterilization for women has been approved in the United States: the Essure method. In this procedure, two metal coils are inserted into the fallopian tubes, where they sit like Slinkys. Over time, tissue grows in and around these inserts to completely block the passage of an egg or sperm. Because the coils are inserted through the vagina and the cervix into the inner part of the uterus where the fallopian tubes open up, the procedure requires no incisions, no general anesthesia, and can be done in an office. Three months later, you'll need a pelvic X-ray to make sure that both tubes are completely blocked.

Not every gynecologist is trained in this procedure, so your doctor may have to refer you to another physician.

Pros: Very effective; failure rate is one in five hundred in the first year, and even lower after that.

Cons: Risks include puncturing the uterus, inability to place one or both coils, failure with an increased risk of ectopic pregnancy, irregular bleeding and cramping, and allergic reaction to the coil materials.

Intrauterine Devices

Another option for women who don't want children (or *more* children) is an intrauterine device (IUD). Technically this isn't permanent, since the device has to be replaced after a few years, but it's very effective. I recommend the Mirena IUD, which releases a small amount of progesterone, called levonorgestrel, into the uterus. This produces lower blood levels of progesterone than the birth control pill produces.

Pros: Can be inserted in an in-office procedure and stay in place for five years and is 99 percent effective in preventing pregnancy. Low doses of progesterone can help control heavy menstrual bleeding. (In fact, Mirena is approved for treatment of heavy menstrual bleeding, separate from contraception.) Since it is not uncommon for women in their forties to have irregular periods as they approach menopause, an IUD can kill two birds with one stone.

Cons: A higher risk of ectopic pregnancy if pregnancy does occur, as with the Essure or tubal ligation procedures. Also, with insertion there is a small but real risk of perforating the uterus, in which case the IUD would end up loose in the abdominal cavity, requiring surgical removal. Chance for uterine or pelvic infection, usually occurring one week after the IUD is inserted, which would require treatment with antibiotics, possible hospitalization, and possible removal of the IUD.

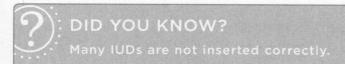

DID YOU KNOW?
Many IUDs are not inserted correctly.

The IUD won't work correctly unless it's placed in the correct position within the uterus. For this reason, you should get an ultrasound within two weeks of placement to make sure it's in the right place.

Vasectomies: To Snip or Not to Snip?

After we had our second child, my husband and I decided our family was complete. My husband decided to have a vasectomy. He felt it was the least he could do, after all I'd gone through with pregnancies and worrying about birth control in the past. Now he recommends it to his patients and to his friends. What a guy!

Rob's in good company. In the United States, an estimated 11–14 percent of men in their thirties and forties have had a vasectomy. More than half a million vasectomies are performed every year. Still, many myths surround this procedure. Here's the truth.

A vasectomy is a minor surgical procedure in which the doctor cuts a tube called the vas deferens, which carries sperm from the testicles, where it mixes with the rest of the semen. Although the man will continue to produce sperm, it will get naturally reabsorbed back into the body (just as it does if a man does not ejaculate). He'll still ejaculate semen, but it won't contain sperm. Thus, no babies.

After a vasectomy, the man needs to either abstain from sex or use condoms for three months after the surgery, and then undergo two semen analyses to make sure that there are no sperm contained in the semen.

Pros: Very effective: Only one in a hundred vasectomies fail within five years of surgery. Can be done in an office setting, with local anesthesia, and only takes about fifteen minutes. Recovery involves ibuprofen, ice, and rest for forty-eight hours.

Cons: Possible long-term scrotal pain, which can occur in up to 15 percent of men.

Many men are worried that the surgery will change their ability to perform sexually. This is a myth! The ability to have an erection and to ejaculate remains unchanged. Some men actually report an *increased* sex drive after vasectomy, due to the more spontaneous and carefree nature of intimacy.

In the end, it's important to know that you have more options for contraception now than ever before. Your choice depends on your age and desires for fertility, so find a doctor who can help you consider them all, not just the ones that he or she can provide.

The New ABCs on STIs

The last time you heard about sexually transmitted infections (STIs) they were probably called STDs (for *sexually transmitted diseases*), or even VD (for *venereal disease*). Many doctors now prefer to call them STIs, because it's a more accurate description than the generic *disease*. We know much more now than we did twenty years ago, and what you don't know about STIs actually *can* hurt you.

By the way, I feel the need to remind you that married women get STIs all the time. At least once every month or two, one of my married patients comes in telling me they've caught their husband having an affair—or even sleeping with prostitutes! Every year, one or two of these women end up with an STI from their cheating spouse. In New Jersey, where I live, this isn't just sad—it's criminal. Giving your spouse an STI after cheating qualifies as criminal assault.

Of course, it's not always the husbands who cheat. Whether you're faithful or not, you need to know how to protect yourself from STIs. Here, I'll brief you on the two most common infections I see in my patients: herpes and human papillomavirus (HPV). These are the ones you're most likely to get, and I want you to know what to do.

GENITAL HERPES

In the United States, one out of every five women ages fourteen to forty-nine has genital herpes. According to the Centers for Disease Control (CDC), the number of Americans with genital herpes increased 30 percent from the late 1970s to the early 1990s, and continues to grow today. Most of these people don't even know they have the virus, which can lay dormant or produce few or no symptoms.

Herpes comes in two forms, HSV-1 and HSV-2, both caused by the herpes simplex virus. HSV-1 usually causes herpes blisters (cold sores) on the lips, and HSV-2 usually causes genital blisters.[1] But really, either form can cause blisters in either location. If someone has a herpes blister on her lip and engages in oral sex, she can pass that virus to her partner genitally. In fact, one study found that women who received oral sex were nine times more likely to become infected with HSV-1 than women who did not.[2]

The symptoms of genital herpes differ from person to person. The classic symptoms (a tingling itch, an ache, throbbing or burning pain, and multiple blisters) may not appear in every woman. If a woman does get symptoms of a first outbreak, they usually occur within two weeks after sexual contact with a partner who has herpes. She may have a fever, and the lymph nodes in the groin may be painful and enlarged, but she might not get blisters and might never suspect herpes.

Not only do symptoms vary, but even herpes tests aren't always accurate. If a blister is fresh, not old and healed, doctors can do a culture on it. Ideally, this is done within the first two to three days of an outbreak. Unfortunately, the test sometimes gives false negatives, so you might have herpes even if the test says otherwise. (False positives, on the other hand, aren't a problem: If you test positive, you definitely have herpes.) Blood tests also have problems because they're not always done correctly. It's best to request a specific test known as HerpeSelect or at least to request that *both* HSV-1 and HSV-2 IgM and IgG antibodies are tested. If there's any question about the results, the test can be repeated in twelve to sixteen weeks (that's how long it takes for the body to produce antibodies in response to the virus).

If you get one of the dreaded positives, you're not alone, and it doesn't make you a bad person. The thing that *would* reflect badly on your character would be not to tell your partner. No matter how painful you find it, you have to discuss your diagnosis with your spouse or partner, not only for his protection, but also because he may already have it (and might have given it to you!). While there is no cure, there *is* safe and effective treatment for herpes. Antiviral therapy, such as the brand-name medication Valtrex, can prevent outbreaks or reduce their duration and severity while decreasing the chance of passing the virus to others. Since the virus can be shed even before actual symptoms or blisters occur, people can be contagious and not know it. Keeping your immune system strong is another important part in reducing outbreaks.

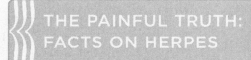

THE PAINFUL TRUTH: FACTS ON HERPES

- One in five women in the United States has genital herpes.
- Herpes may have minimal or no symptoms.
- Herpes can be treated but not cured.
- Herpes can be passed even when there are no visible blisters or sores.

HUMAN PAPILLOMAVIRUS

Human papillomavirus (HPV), which causes genital warts, is the single most common STI. By the age of fifty, a whopping 50–80 percent of women have been exposed to HPV via intimate skin-to-skin contact or sexual intercourse. It's tough to avoid: After all, there are more than a hundred different strains of HPV. Some cause abnormal Pap smears, genital warts, or cervical cancer, but the virus is also a leading cause of oral/throat, penile, vulvar, vaginal, and anal cancers.

The good news is that 90 percent of people exposed to HPV will clear the virus from their bodies within two to three years. Many will never even know they had it. But for approximately thirty-two thousand people a year diagnosed with HPV-related cancers, this virus can be deadly.

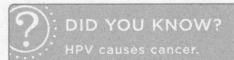

DID YOU KNOW?
HPV causes cancer.

Every year in the United States, thousands of people are diagnosed with HPV-related cancers, including:

- 3,700 cases of vulvar cancer
- 1,000 cases of vaginal cancer
- 1,000 cases of penile cancer
- 4,400 cases of anal cancer
- 12,000 cases of cervical cancer

HPV Testing

Many gynecologists routinely screen for HPV, but not all do, so ask your doctor to do so. If you test positive for HPV, that doesn't mean you got it recently. You might have gotten it years earlier.

Of course, if the virus causes genital warts, you'll know. They're ugly, but not necessarily painful. Treatments include acid, removal by laser or scalpel, or immune-modulating medications.

The best ways to reduce your exposure to HPV include limiting the number of sexual partners and practicing safe sex. Condoms help, but they're not 100 percent effective, because they don't cover every millimeter of skin. If you're under twenty-six you can get vaccinated against HPV, but the vaccine hasn't been approved for people in their late twenties or older.

PROTECTING YOURSELF

One of the very best parts of keeping your body beautiful is getting to enjoy sex and intimacy, whether it's thrilling, naughty, and new or loving, warm, and familiar (or all of those!). Talking about STIs might put a damper on that, but there's a lot you can do to keep your next adventure safe and empowering.

If You're Dating

Get tested. Ask your doctor to do a full STI panel on you (and ask your partner to get one done, too!). This includes blood tests for hepatitis B and C, HIV, syphilis, and cervical cultures for chlamydia and gonorrhea for you (urine cultures for chlamydia and gonorrhea for him). Most doctors don't include routine herpes blood tests because the results can be so inconclusive, but talk with your doctor about it.

Repeat the tests in several months. Many viruses have latency periods, so a person can be infected and not show any positive results. For this reason, staggered or repeat testing is a good idea. Repeat the tests after three, six, and twelve months. Keep in mind, however, that if you or your partner has sex with someone else during that time, you may be exposed and the test results will mean nothing.

Use condoms. Condoms are the only way, besides abstinence, to prevent the spread of many STIs. But they're not perfect. As I mentioned above, they slip, leak, or break 17 percent of the time, and you may not even know it. To avoid failure, make sure your partner is using the right size condom in the right manner (leaving space at the end for semen and holding it at the rimmed end until it can be safely removed after ejaculation). You also need to know what to do if one breaks. Not only is pregnancy a possibility, but so is infection. If a condom breaks, call your gynecologist within twenty-four to forty-eight hours.

In the end, the most important thing you can do for yourself sexually is to remember this: Sex doesn't end at forty. It doesn't have to end at all. Understanding your contraceptive options and knowing the facts about STIs are important parts of making sure your sex life stays healthy, happy, and beautiful in the decades ahead.

Great Expectations

Pregnancy for Grown-ups

Congratulations! You've peed on the little wand and you've seen the pink plus sign! Or you're hoping to see it soon! Either way, you're in good company: Nearly 10 percent of first births today are to women over age thirty-five. That's a huge change from our mothers' generation. Back in 1970, only one in a hundred first births were to women over thirty-five.[1] Although we obstetricians will still label you as AMA (advanced maternal age), it doesn't seem so advanced at all these days. In fact, sometimes I think we should call it SMA (sophisticated maternal age). While you'll probably hear a lot about the risks of pregnancy when you're over thirty-five (which I'll tell you about in this chapter), there are real advantages, too, including social, financial, and psychological security and stability that you might not have had in your twenties. In short, sometimes the thirties and forties are the *best* time to have a baby.

Since there are lots of fabulous books on pregnancy out there, I'll only highlight the topics most important for moms-to-be in their thirties or forties, including fertility treatments, specific risks of mature pregnancies, and the pros and cons of C-sections.

The Science of ART (Assisted Reproductive Technologies)

Of the 4.3 million babies born in the United States every year, approximately forty thousand of them are born with assisted reproductive technology (ART). In other words, their parents had some medical help getting pregnant. During our lifetimes, advances in fertility sciences have made making babies very big business indeed.

Typically, doctors suspect you may have fertility issues if you've tried to become pregnant with no luck for one year. But because fertility begins to decline around age thirty-five, it's not uncommon for women in their mid-thirties (and their doctors) to start infertility testing and treatment prior to the one-year mark. After all, the clock is ticking on those eggs. Fortunately, your regular gynecologist can do a lot of this testing before you move on to an infertility specialist. Here's a quick rundown on the typical tests you'll go through.

Semen analysis: Up to 30 percent of infertility problems lie with the man. The semen may contain too few sperm, sperm that don't swim well, or sperm that die too quickly. For this reason, one of the very first tests a doctor will suggest is a semen analysis.

Blood tests: Your doctor will order a blood draw to make sure you have the right levels of thyroid hormone, testosterone, progesterone, follicle stimulating hormone (or FSH, which promotes egg growth), and luteinizing hormone (or LH, which triggers ovulation).

Saline sonogram: Not to be confused with a regular sonogram,

which you'll get often once you become pregnant, the saline sonogram is a special type of pelvic sonogram or ultrasound in which
a small amount of saline (salt water) is injected into the uterine
cavity. The solution pushes the walls of the uterus apart from each
other. The water appears black on an ultrasound, and you can see
an outline of the endometrial cavity. Any polyps or fibroids, which
can interfere with the implantation of any embryo, will appear
silhouetted in white. Because any defects in the lining of the uterine cavity can potentially cause problems, this is one of the first
tests that an infertility specialist or thorough gynecologist will do.

Hysterosalpingogram (HSG): This is a special kind of X-ray that
shows whether the fallopian tubes are open or blocked. Usually
done during the first week of a period and always *after* a negative
pregnancy test, a small amount of dye is pushed into the uterus
and into the fallopian tubes while a pelvic X-ray is taken. A good
result shows "fill and spill"—the dye moves up the fallopian
tubes, meaning there's a clear path for the sperm to meet and fertilize the egg, and then travel into the uterus. A word of caution:
If your tubes are completely or partially blocked, this test can be
uncomfortable or painful. If you feel pain during the test, don't
be afraid to speak up and tell the technician.

Ovulation tests: With conception, as with comedy, timing is everything. Your doctor will help you track whether you're ovulating regularly. If you have a regular cycle, you ovulate fourteen
days before your period starts. So, if you got your period on day
28 of your cycle, that means you ovulated on day 14. If you got
your period on day 30, you ovulated on day 16. To get pregnant,
you need to have sex when you're ovulating, so tracking ovulation
is important. Fortunately, it's fairly simple to do. Your basal body
temperature goes up and cervical mucus increases and becomes
more stretchy, so you can track those things yourself. You can also
buy an over-the-counter ovulation predictor kit, where you pee

on a stick every day. This indicates when urinary levels of LH rise. Your doctor can also check your blood levels of FSH on day 3 of your cycle to check your ovarian reserve, or roughly how many eggs are left in your ovaries.

FERTILITY TREATMENTS

If you and your ob-gyn decide that infertility treatments are in order, remember that even with today's remarkable technologies it takes time to conceive. There's no quick fix, but there's a wide variety of treatments. Just a few common ones include:

Clomid: This is a pill you take for five days during your cycle to jump-start ovulation. It's often the first line of fertility treatment, since it has few side effects, but it won't work if the problem is something physical, like blocked fallopian tubes. Other medications can also induce ovulation, including Metformin, often prescribed for women with polycystic ovarian syndrome (PCOS).

Repronex or other shots: Some shots containing FSH or other medications can induce ovulation. You give yourself these shots on certain days of your cycle, often in preparation for artificial insemination or in vitro fertilization (IVF).

Surgery: In the case of blocked fallopian tubes, a simple laparoscopic procedure can clear out blockages and permit eggs to travel to the uterus for fertilization. Sometimes, surgery to tie off fallopian tubes will also be used before in vitro fertilization, because blocked or damaged tubes often secrete an inflammatory substance that decreases IVF success rates.

Artificial insemination: After inducing ovulation with medications, your doctor will inject sperm from your partner or a donor into your uterus to fertilize your eggs. This is also called intrauterine insemination (IUI).

In vitro fertilization (IVF): Your doctor will remove your eggs and fertilize them in vitro with your partner's sperm (donor eggs or sperm can also be used). Later, the embryos will be implanted in your uterus.

Donor eggs: I suggest this option to women who are unlikely or unable to use their own eggs to conceive, because of a variety of factors that may include age, quality of eggs, premature menopause, or chemotherapy resulting in infertility. In this process, a woman selects a donor who has agreed to provide eggs, often from a registry of egg donors, which may then be fertilized with her husband's sperm in vitro, then implanted in her own uterus.

Surrogacy: If a woman's uterus will not support a pregnancy, she doesn't have a uterus anymore, or she is physically unwilling or unable to carry a pregnancy, she may choose to hire a surrogate mother, who can gestate an embryo created either through IVF using the biological mother's eggs and father's sperm, or with donor eggs. The laws surrounding surrogacy differ by state, and the process is an expensive one, but it can be helpful to women in their forties and beyond who want children.

Adoption: Despite many heartbreaking stories of long waits and disappointments with adoption, many parents have very positive experiences with adoption, both domestic and international.

For more information on these options and for terrific support for all infertility issues, visit Resolve, the National Infertility Association, at www.resolve.org.

RISKS OF INFERTILITY TREATMENTS

With so many options available today, the end message is clear and hopeful: If you want children in your life, you'll have them, one way or another. But whatever options you pursue, you'll need to be aware of the risks.

Miscarriages: About 16 percent of pregnancies, whether they used ART or not, end in miscarriage. While common, miscarriage—and especially repeated miscarriages—can be heartbreaking.

Multiples: Anyone who's watched *Kate Plus 8* knows that IVF or other infertility treatments bring an increased rate of multiples (usually twins or triplets). With natural conception, only one to two pregnancies in a hundred will yield twins or triplets. But if you receive infertility treatments, your chances rise to thirty-two in a hundred. Any multiple birth carries a higher risk to mother and babies, particularly of preterm delivery. A whopping sixty-three out of a hundred twins are born prematurely; ninety-five of a hundred triplets are early. These babies risk lifelong complications. In general, the risk of preterm delivery across all ART methods is 12 percent, which is similar to the risk for a singleton.[2]

Birth defects: There continues to be debate in the field about whether babies conceived through IVF have a higher rate of birth defects. Some studies have shown an association, but it is unclear whether this might stem from the ART process or from the underlying infertility issues. At this point, you should talk with your doctor about the risk of birth defects if you're considering infertility treatments.

You're Pregnant: Now What?

Through whatever means, you've gotten pregnant! Congratulations! Chances are you'll sail through pregnancy. But it's important to know that women over thirty-five are at slightly higher risk for the general complications of pregnancy, including preterm labor, abruption of the placenta, gestational diabetes, and preeclampsia. We don't know exactly why the risks are higher, but we do know that the human female body is meant to reproduce in the early twenties (even if our brains, emotions, and wallets are better suited for kids later on!). In our mid-thirties and beyond, the baby-making machinery still works, but in some women, those mechanisms can be a little more delicate, so to speak. So we obstetricians tend to watch our older pregnant women just a little more closely than we do our patients in their twenties (and trust me, we watch them pretty darn closely, too!). I like to see my "mature" pregnant patients a little more often than patients in their twenties. It differs from patient to patient, but I usually see my patients in their thirties and beyond every two weeks starting around 28 weeks, and then weekly after 34 weeks.

Many OBs will do a few extra sonograms on a mother over thirty-five to monitor growth of the fetus and levels of amniotic fluid. They may also do a non-stress test in the third trimester. This is a very simple, noninvasive test where a fetal heart rate monitor is put around the mother's abdomen for twenty to thirty minutes. We measure the baby's movements and heart rate, and look for signs that the baby is receiving enough oxygen. The heart rate of a healthy fetus increases when it moves, and stays steady when it's still or sleeping.

GESTATIONAL DIABETES

Pregnant women over thirty-five are at higher risk for gestational diabetes mellitus (GDM), which affects as many as four hundred thousand pregnancies a year.

When I did my OB-GYN residency, I was fortunate enough to be trained by the world's expert in GDM, Dr. Oded Langer. Later, when I went into private practice, I was shocked to see that many experienced OBs were still managing pregnant women as they'd been trained to ten, twenty, or thirty years earlier. Proper GDM diagnosis and treatment can literally mean the difference between a healthy pregnancy and delivery and a compromised one, so I want you to have the inside scoop on current trends in managing patients with GDM.

In GDM, a mother's body suffers a temporary inability to process glucose. In response, her pancreas churns out more insulin than normal. This promotes an unhealthy rate of growth in all fetal organs, including the heart, liver, and pancreas, and stresses the baby's blood vessels and the mother's placenta. Untreated, GDM can lead to either a high or low birth weight, premature delivery, an increased chance of cesarean delivery, and a slightly increased risk of fetal or neonatal death.

You're at higher risk of GDM if you're over thirty-five, if you've had GDM in a previous pregnancy, have a strong history of diabetes, or have polycystic ovarian syndrome (PCOS). You're also at elevated risk if you're African-American, Hispanic, Asian, or American Indian.

Testing for GDM

The standard time for a GDM screening is between weeks 24 and 28 of pregnancy. However, if one of my patients has any risk factors, I test her earlier, during the first trimester, around 8–12 weeks. If she passes, I'll test again in the second trimester. The first trimester is a critical time for organ formation, so it's wise to find out early if there's any degree of insulin resistance. The test is a simple blood test, taken one hour after drinking a glucose liquid.

Many OBs have their patients fast the night before this test, but that's actually not necessary. I recommend having a sandwich on whole-wheat bread the day before to give your body a decent base of good carbs that will help keep your glucose and insulin in good balance before the test.

If your results are slightly abnormal (above 135 but below 140), you may or may not be asked to do a three-hour follow-up test. Personally, when my patients show only slightly abnormal levels, I don't always do the three-hour test. Instead, I recommend that they start eating and exercising as though they were diabetic. I have them limit their sugars and simple carbohydrates while exercising more, both of which help stabilize blood glucose levels. Then I follow them closely for the rest of the pregnancy, since GDM can present itself at any time.

If your glucose levels are more elevated on the first test (over 140), you'll have to do the three-hour glucose challenge. In this test, you fast the night before, have blood drawn, drink a stronger version of the glucose cocktail, and have your blood rechecked every hour for three hours. Your numbers should be below 95 on the first draw, 180 at hour one, 155 at hour two, and 140 at hour three.[3]

If the fasting value is abnormal or if two other numbers are abnormal, you qualify as a gestational diabetic. In my opinion, too many OBs allow a loose interpretation of these numbers and aren't aggressive enough in treating GDM. I believe that swiftly addressing diet and behavior, and possibly prescribing medication, can make a major difference for mothers and babies at risk for GDM.

Fortunately, GDM is a common condition and most ob-gyns are well versed in its treatment—you may not have to see a high-risk OB. However, every obstetrician will have his or her own style of management, so talk with yours about how they follow their GDM patients.

I see my patients with GDM every week to monitor their sugars, their blood pressure (since having GDM increases the risk of preeclampsia), and fetal growth and well-being. I may recommend that they meet with a nutritionist for dietary guidance, and start testing their own blood sugar at home with a finger-prick glucometer first thing in the morning and two hours after eating. I recommend ultrasounds every four weeks to assess the growth of the baby and the amount of amniotic fluid. Beginning at 34 weeks, I recommend fetal non-stress tests to make sure the baby's okay. Some patients may require medication: Pregnant women with GDM can now be placed on a pill called Metformin, and may not necessarily require insulin, to control their blood sugar.

RISKS OF GESTATIONAL DIABETES

- fetal macrosomia (larger baby)
- fetal growth restriction (smaller baby)
- fetal metabolic abnormalities after birth
- increased risk of C-section
- increased risk of shoulder dystocia (baby getting stuck during delivery)
- increased risk of preeclampsia (high blood pressure in pregnancy)
- increased risk for the mother of type 2 diabetes in the future

As many as 50 percent of women who have had diabetes in pregnancy will become diabetic in the years or decades following that pregnancy.[4] For this reason, getting tested again *after* you deliver is vitally important for your health. National guidelines recommend testing all women who had gestational diabetes approximately six to twelve weeks after pregnancy. This can be simply done with a fasting glucose test.

To C or Not to C: C-sections, Inductions, and Elective Delivery

The first law of delivery: The one day you *know* you won't deliver on is your official due date. In reality, only about 5 percent of babies spontaneously arrive on their due dates. But wouldn't it be great if you could plan exactly when you'd go into labor and put it in your date book? Some women are doing that through elective delivery, a topic that's gotten lots of media attention lately. Each side has its pros and cons.

Certainly there are times when it's medically advisable to induce labor. The mom may have high blood pressure, bleeding, infection, or be taking certain medications like blood thinners that require a controlled delivery. Or maybe the mom has had two babies already, has had fast deliveries, and lives an hour away from the hospital. If she's not induced at the hospital, she may very well deliver that baby at home on the sofa! Sometimes, the baby needs labor to be induced, because it has an abnormal heart tracing, it doesn't seem to be moving or growing, or it has a birth defect that requires sophisticated care immediately after delivery (where teams of physicians need to be assembled and ready to perform surgery). None of these instances are really *elective* reasons for induction, because inducing is medically necessary for the good of the mother or baby.

With true elective induction, a woman or her doctor simply decides to deliver the baby at a certain point because they *want* to. Why not? It's a free country, right? True. But there are risks with inductions, including an elevated chance of C-section if the cervix is not ready for labor. In addition, the baby's well-being depends on the proper timing of delivery. When we date a pregnancy and determine your due date, we calculate from the first day of your last period before conception. But even with sonograms to confirm the due date, this dating can easily be off by a week or so. What's the big deal? The baby's lungs may not be ready to breathe and complications can ensue. National guidelines advise against induction before 39 weeks unless an amniocentesis has determined the baby's lungs are mature enough to breathe. In my opinion, elective induction is a step to take with great caution.

TOO POSH TO PUSH? ELECTIVE C-SECTIONS

In the United States, the overall C-section rate is approximately 30 percent and has increased dramatically over the past decade. Why? More patients are requesting it. But physicians are also afraid of being sued if things go wrong during a vaginal birth.

Elective deliveries are also on the rise in other parts of the world. In China, the C-section rate is 60 percent, and in parts of South America having one's baby by C-section is considered a privilege of the elite. In many regions, women believe that sparing their pelvic floor the trauma of childbirth will protect their sexual function in the future. In some circles, this practice of elective C-section is often referred to as being "too posh to push."

Because C-sections are so common, it's easy to forget that a cesarean is a *major* operation. As one of my esteemed colleagues is fond of saying, "This isn't like getting your nails done."

In the United States, where we have access to excellent anesthesia, sterile operating rooms, great neonatal medical care, and blood transfusion services, the risk of dying after a C-section is relatively low. Still, the possibility needs to be taken seriously, as do all the risks of C-sections.

In general, birth via C-section is safer than vaginal birth for the baby and riskier for the mother. But babies still face risks. Babies delivered abdominally by C-section have a higher incidence of temporary respiratory issues than do babies who are born vaginally. In addition, even though the risk of a shoulder dystocia (where the baby's shoulder gets stuck under the pelvic bone during a vaginal delivery) is much lower, it *is* possible to have difficulty getting the baby out abdominally, and this too can result in nerve injury affecting the baby's arm.

The risks to the mother during a C-section involve injury or damage to other parts of the pelvic anatomy (like a bladder injury), infection (either in the pelvic area or superficially on the surface of the skin), and anesthesia complications (although this last is very rare). Also, having one C-section increases the risk of uterine rupture in future pregnancies, along with increasing the risk of problems with the placenta in the future.

Given a thorough and comprehensive discussion of all the risks and benefits of elective C-sections, many physicians today feel that this should be a woman's choice.

The problem, as I see it, is that too many physicians do not present an unbiased view of the pros and cons. In addition, some OBs charge more for a C-section than for a vaginal delivery. This never made sense to me, considering that it takes far less time to do a C-section (typically thirty minutes or less) than a vaginal delivery (which often takes hours).

If you are considering requesting an elective C-section, here are the questions you should ask your doctor.

- What are the risks to me?
- What are the risks to my baby?
- What does this mean for future pregnancies?
- Is there a cost difference (either affecting me or my insurance)?

Also, if you've decided that this is your last child and you're considering having your tubes tied, ask if that can be done after the delivery, since the incision is already made.

SECOND TIME AROUND?
VAGINAL BIRTH AFTER CESAREAN

Some OBs and their patients believe that once you've had one C-section, all your later babies need to be delivered abdominally as well. But that's not actually true. In fact, we now know that having a vaginal birth after cesarean (VBAC) can be safer than having another C-section. But, as usual, it's not a black-and-white issue. The big worry with a VBAC is the rare but potentially deadly rupture of the uterus. A woman who has already had a C-section and tries a VBAC has a 1.6 in a thousand risk of a uterine rupture before labor even starts. If labor starts spontaneously, the risk rises to 5.2 per thousand women, and to 7.7 per thousand when labor is induced with the drug Pitocin. The risk can go as high as 24.5 in a thousand women when labor is induced with prosta-glandins (commonly known by the brand name Cervidil).[5]

These risks are low, but they're very real—and taking risks with the life and death of a mother and her baby is not something that most obstetricians like to do. If the uterus ruptures, the baby can die or be severely disabled for life, and the mother can hemorrhage and require a blood transfusion and/or an emergency hysterectomy.

That said, delivering vaginally and avoiding a repeat C-section can be done safely and with less risk to the mother than that presented by major surgery. Talk about this option with your doctor, and if necessary, get a second opinion.

When you consider a VBAC, your doctor will ask what led to the first C-section. If the baby got stuck, your cervix stopped dilating, or you had a uterine rupture, those problems may recur and, in general, you're not a good risk for VBAC. But if your first C-section was due to fetal distress, a placenta problem, or a multiple birth, your chances of a suc-cessful VBAC are good. See the chart below for a simplified breakdown.

CHANCES OF A SUCCESSFUL VBAC

Your chances of a successful VBAC depend on why you had your first C-section.

Reason for C-section	Chance of Successful VBAC
Fetal distress	Good
Breech	Depends
Fever/infection	Good
Baby got stuck during pushing	Poor

Cervix stopped dilating	Poor
Bleeding/placental problem	Good
Maternal issue (high blood pressure, etc.)	Good
Uterine rupture	Poor
Twins	Good

If you decide to try a VBAC, don't be surprised to learn that procedures differ from one hospital and doctor to another, including how the baby will be monitored, the type of anesthesia given, whether or not the OB will be present for the entire duration of the labor, and whether or not any drugs such as Pitocin will be used to start or assist the labor process. In my case, I want continuous fetal monitoring when attempting a VBAC. When possible, I prefer to apply a monitor directly to the baby's scalp, so we know for sure that we're seeing the baby's heart rate, not the mother's, on the monitor.

In addition, I believe that epidural anesthesia is the safest choice for the mother and the baby when trying a VBAC. This way, in case an emergency C-section becomes necessary, the mother does not need to be put to sleep, creating a safer situation for her and her baby.

Because the uterus is much more likely to rupture when prostaglandins are used to induce labor, and slightly higher when Pitocin is used, I prefer to use no uterine stimulating drugs during a VBAC. (But plenty of other OBs *do* use them, safely.)

Finally, I stay with my patients for the entire duration of their labor when they are attempting a VBAC. Though emergencies are uncommon, every minute counts when they do occur, so I prefer to be right there throughout the entire labor. I tend to err on the side of caution: If anything at all crops up that's out of the ordinary, including a fever, the need for Pitocin or a vacuum delivery, or the presence of meconium (fetal stool), I will perform a repeat C-section. But bear in mind, this is my own individual style. Your doctor may have a different, equally safe and valid approach. The important thing is that you ask enough questions so you know what to expect.

Special Delivery?

Many of my mature patients already have older children, excited to meet their new little brother or sister. Some patients today invite their children into the delivery room, but this only applies to a vaginal delivery. Visitors are not permitted at a C-section or other major surgery.

If you choose to have your children in the delivery room, be aware that it might frighten children younger than twelve or thirteen to see their mom go through labor. (Some hospitals will not allow younger children in the delivery room.) Be sure to ask your kids if they *really want* to be there, explain that they may find some of what they see disturbing, and have a backup plan for them if they feel sick or frightened. The last thing you want while you're pushing is to be worried about the child standing next to your bed, as well as the child you're delivering. The second-to-last thing you want is for your nurse and/or doctor to be distracted by another child in the room who may be fainting or vomiting! Think about all these scenarios before you invite your older children to witness the delivery. After all, even if they can't be in the room for the actual birth, many hospitals will allow them to see the new baby within an hour of delivery.

Breast-feeding: Feast or Beast?

Everybody knows that breast-feeding is great for your child's health. Not everybody knows that it can be a real beast to master. When I had my first baby, I thought breast-feeding would be a breeze. After all, I was a medical student. I had breasts, he had a mouth—what could go wrong?

I couldn't have been more mistaken. My son had difficulty latching on; I used nipple shields to ease the initial pain (which turned out to be a mistake for me); I didn't produce enough milk. Before I knew it, he had lost more than 10 percent of his birth weight. I ended up feeding him with formula, and then nursing him, for three months. Breast-feeding just never really went well with baby number one. I felt I'd failed at a basic maternal practice, until my ob-gyn, Dr. Ben Pascario, reassured me. "The important word in *breast-feeding* is *feeding*. Feed your baby the best way you can and be happy that he's eating," he said. He was absolutely right. There's more than enough guilt to go around for mothers without piling one more thing on the list.

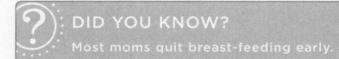

DID YOU KNOW?
Most moms quit breast-feeding early.

Recent studies show that although 77 percent of mothers try breast-feeding their babies, only 36 percent are still at it six months later.[6] The American Association of Pediatricians recommends that babies be breast-fed for a year.

Still, with my second baby, I was determined to try again. While pregnant, I bought books, equipment, and pumps, had phone numbers for lactation consultants, took classes in the hospital . . . you get the picture. This time, things were very different. My daughter latched on immediately, like she was the one who'd been training for it, and I made enough milk to feed a small village. I used a double electric breast pump at night if she was sleeping to store it up, to stimulate more milk production, and to fully drain each breast after she had nursed. Same two breasts, totally different experiences!

Personally, I feel great sympathy for moms who have trouble breast-feeding, especially today, when even complete strangers look askance at us when we whip out a bottle instead of a breast. There's no question that medically, breast-feeding's benefits far outweigh any downsides. Breast-fed babies have stronger immune systems, fewer ear infections, lower rates of diabetes, a lower risk of sudden infant death syndrome (SIDS), and may have a higher IQ by age eight than babies who don't receive breast milk.[7] Moms benefit from breast-feeding, too. They have lower risks of breast cancer and they lose the baby weight more quickly, since breast-feeding burns a huge number of calories. And it's a lovely opportunity to bond with your baby.

But it's not for everyone. Some babies don't latch on, some babies have reflux or other problems that make it difficult, and some moms can't tolerate the initial pain (though some women don't find it painful at all). So forget what TV celebrities or strangers on the bus tell you when they offer unsolicited advice. I tell my patients to breast-feed if they can to reap the enormous benefits. But if they can't, don't dwell on it.

MASTITIS WHILE BREAST-FEEDING

Some breast-feeding moms develop an infection called mastitis, which occurs when bacteria from the skin or the baby's mouth enter the breast through the nipple. You may feel extremely sick, run a temperature above 101 degrees, or have shaking chills, red streaks on one or both breasts, and breast tenderness or swelling. On very rare occasions, I've admitted patients to the ICU with mastitis that spread through the body and produced septic shock.

If caught early, mastitis is easily treated with oral antibiotics and warm soaks to the breast. While many women think they need to stop breast-feeding if they have mastitis, that's actually the worst thing to do. The milk will build up pressure and cause engorgement in the breast, making the infection more severe.

MASTITIS SYMPTOMS

- High fever (over 101 degrees)
- Red streaks on the breast
- Breast pain
- Hard, tender area on the breast
- Chills
- Feeling overall sick
- Visible pus coming from the nipple

Your Body Bountiful

In the end, pregnancy is an absolutely unique time in a woman's life. The beauty of pregnancy in your thirties and early forties is that you're probably much better equipped, emotionally and psychologically, to handle the challenges. Take comfort in your maturity and, whether you love being pregnant or hate it, remember to pause and appreciate the wonders that your beautiful body can show you.

Hormones

The Truth About Hormone Imbalances, Menopause, and Hormone Replacement Therapy

lmost every single day in my medical practice, a patient comes in worried about a long list of vague symptoms. The list often includes:

- mental fog: being distracted, forgetful, or not focused
- moodiness: having rapid swings from feeling fine to hysterically crying or being short-tempered
- disturbed sleep
- change in body weight (usually a gain)
- low energy
- change in hair patterns (either thinning or in some cases more body hair)
- change in skin (adult acne, dry skin)
- low libido
- hot flashes
- general feeling of being unwell

I always ask what my patients think might be causing the symptoms, because a person's intuition can be very accurate. Nine times out of ten, they say, "I think my hormones are out of whack."

I understand why they say this. Hormones have received a lot of media attention lately, and indeed, sometimes hormone imbalances *do* cause serious problems, including diabetes and Addison's disease. Sometimes the symptoms I listed above can result from a hormone imbalance. But all of these symptoms might also be explained by a wide variety of other causes—medical, social, or environmental—ranging from medication side effects to sleep deprivation. It certainly doesn't help that these signs are very subjective: One woman's low energy day may be another woman's high octane moment. These problems aren't black-and-white like blood pressure, which is either elevated or not. There are a few hormonal conditions that can be easily diagnosed and treated, including some I discuss below, but in general, much more research needs to be done on hormones and their health effects.

Until that happens, so-called hormonal doctors out there will offer to treat women with unproven therapies for conditions that are not medically recognized. These doctors are different from reputable endocrinologists, who are board-certified physicians specializing in recognized hormonal conditions. Instead, some doctors blame *everything* on hormonal imbalances and even develop their own treatments that aren't tested or approved. I don't think it's right to do this: It's emotionally and intellectually misleading to blame a collection of symptoms on hormonal imbalances that have not been studied. To treat these conditions with unresearched therapies exposes women to real risks and side effects. The truth is, there is usually not one hormone to blame for these symptoms, but a much more complex physiology underlying the problems.

Don't get me wrong; I do take the symptoms above very seriously. When a patient thinks she has a hormonal imbalance, I know very likely *something* is out of balance in her health. But I believe in taking a holistic approach, examining all the factors that could cause each symptom, and often recommending small changes over time.

Hormones in Action

Before we go deeper into the controversial topic of hormonal imbalance, you need a good understanding of hormones in general. Hormones are substances that are either made in our bodies or produced synthetically to resemble those made in our bodies. Either way, they control the performance or output of an organ or body system. They're like messengers, carrying a signal to another part of the body or to a body system to either speed up or slow down, or to make more of something or less of it. They're the drill sergeants that shout orders to the army.

But there's more than one army. There are many separate systems in the body controlled by different hormones. One set of hormones controls reproduction, menstruation, and pregnancy; another deals with your immune system and inflammation; one regulates your appetite and metabolism; another controls your fight-or-flight stress response. And there are more! You can see that simply saying "You have a hormonal imbalance" isn't so simple after all. That's like saying "There's weather outside!" Are you talking about a heat wave or a blizzard?

Common Hormonal Imbalances

A few hormonal imbalances, including diabetes, hypothyroidism, and Addison's disease, are fairly easy to diagnose and to treat. The confusion arises when someone doesn't fit the criteria for diagnosis with one of these common problems.

DIABETES

Diabetes is probably the best-known example of a hormonal imbalance. In type 1 diabetes, the body doesn't produce enough of the hormone insulin to process the glucose from the food that we eat. In type 2 diabetes, the insulin that *is* made is too weak or insufficient to carry out efficient glucose metabolism. In both types, the result is an excess of sugar in the blood, which over time damages blood vessels throughout the body.

HYPOTHYROIDISM

Hypothyroidism occurs when the thyroid does not produce enough of its important hormones. Symptoms can include many of those listed at the beginning of the chapter (fatigue or sluggishness, unexplained weight gain, depression) plus constipation, puffiness in the face, a hoarse voice, or pain and stiffness in your joints or muscles.

Hypothyroidism, which is more common in women over fifty than in younger women, can be diagnosed by testing the blood levels of two hormones, thyroid-stimulating hormone (TSH) and thyroxine. Once diagnosed, hypothyroidism is easily treated with either synthetic or natural hormones.

ADDISON'S DISEASE

Addison's disease is an imbalance of the adrenal gland, which produces cortisol (the stress hormone), adrenaline, noradrenaline also known as norepinephrine (the fight-or-flight hormone), aldosterone (which helps regulate blood pressure), and 50 percent of the testosterone that circulates in women's bodies. Addison's disease causes fatigue, chronic diarrhea, loss of appetite, weight loss, and other symptoms, and can be treated with corticosteroids.

Gray Areas

It's very tempting to look at symptoms that are common in these diseases above and assume that, even if tests don't show you have the imbalance, hormones must be at play in some way. For this reason, alternative practitioners or laypeople sometimes come up with unofficial diagnoses. For instance, much attention has been paid to "adrenal fatigue," which is *not* an official medical term or condition. It's a label that alternative practitioners designed to refer to symptoms that resemble the effects of a sluggish adrenal gland, but fall short of the full-blown Addison's disease criteria. Practitioners who believe in this condition feel that the adrenal gland can become "worn out" from chronic stress and therefore doesn't produce enough of the important hormones you need to feel your best—and yet *does* produce enough of them to evade the official diagnosis of Addison's disease.

I'm not saying this condition doesn't exist. This reasoning may, in fact, have some truth to it. I *am* saying that more research needs to be done. Until we know more, my advice to patients is to proceed with caution where any proposed treatment is concerned. Many unregulated, unstudied, over-the-counter supplements are marketed to people suffering from this unrecognized condition. These supplements can be dangerous and can distract both the patient and a medically qualified physician from finding the true cause of these bothersome symptoms.

The same dilemma can exist with almost every hormonal system in the body. Women always ask me to check their hormones to get to the bottom of their symptoms. But it's just not that simple. Hormonal levels vary hour to hour and day to day. Yes, tests can rule out certain conditions like Addison's or hypothyroidism. But for hormones including progesterone, estrogen, and testosterone, there is *no* accepted protocol for matching blood test results with therapy. In other words, in gynecology, we don't give X amount of progesterone to a woman with a blood level of Y. Some hormonal practitioners believe you can test salivary hormone levels and create remedies based on those tests, but this has *never* been studied with scientific rigor.

I believe more research on hormones should be done so we can discover if there is any plausible truth to treating women with different doses and formulations of various hormones. But until that research exists, treating patients for unproven hormonal imbalances, with unapproved therapies, is pure speculation.

HOW I TREAT SUSPECTED HORMONAL IMBALANCES

So what about the many, many women of all ages who just "don't feel right" and have the very common and vague symptoms I listed at the beginning of the chapter that may indeed have hormonal origins, but aren't official conditions? I feel that the smartest, soundest medical approach is to evaluate the patient, head to toe, and exclude the most common and the most dangerous possible causes first. This involves a complete physical exam, running general blood tests, and reviewing all medications, supplements, and possible environmental factors that could be contributing to the symptoms.

If no obvious cause is found, my next step is to examine my patients' diets. All too often, people deprive their bodies of the nutrients and fuel necessary for top physical functioning.

Next, I target my patients' sleep habits. As I mentioned earlier, many, maybe most, women are sleep-deprived and don't even know it. Hormones would be an easier explanation in some ways than sleep deprivation, especially if the condition could be treated with a simple pill. It's not easy to revamp our behavior and lifestyle so we can get more sleep. But every single symptom I listed above can be caused by too little shut-eye (and, by the way, inadequate sleep can subtly affect our body's hormonal balance).

Finally, I focus on fitness and exercise. Your beautiful body wants to move and needs to be active. When we exercise, natural feel-good chemicals (endorphins) are produced. Every blood vessel in the body reaps the benefits, which in turn can improve feeling and function in the brain, digestive tract, metabolism, and reproductive tract.

Again, I'm not saying diet, exercise, and sleep can cure every problem, and I would never dismiss a patient's symptoms. But my own experience shows that many of these complaints go away with close attention to diet, exercise, and sleep habits.

Hormones and Menopause

Of course, there *is* one time in your life when a major hormone system rebalances itself: menopause.

At some point in time, every woman will go through menopause. The age of menopause varies from woman to woman, depending on factors including your family history, genetics, and other issues. Smoking can bring on early menopause, as can some chronic diseases and some cancer treatments.

The average age of menopause in the United States is fifty-one, but these changes can start even as early as your thirties or occur as late as your mid-fifties. The key hormonal events that define menopause involve a decrease in the amount of estrogen, progesterone, and testosterone made by your ovaries. (Yes, your ovaries produce testosterone!)

When you were still a fetus in your mother's uterus, your ovaries contained between 7 and 20 million eggs! At birth, that number dropped to 1 to 2 million, and by the time you had your first period, you had about three hundred thousand eggs left. It sounds like more than enough—and it is. Over the course of your reproductive life, you'll release about three hundred to four hundred eggs. At some point, your ovaries start to run out of eggs and they approach the end of the reproductive stage of their life.

As your ovaries get tired and less productive, they produce less estrogen, less progesterone, and less testosterone. As the production of these hormones goes down, the level of another hormone, called follicle stimulating hormone (FSH), goes up, indicating that the pituitary is trying to work harder to get the ovaries to do the same work they used to do. Another hormone, called inhibin, begins to drop, which allows the FSH level to increase. As these hormone levels change, and sometimes slightly before, women may begin to have a variety of symptoms, from hot flashes to moodiness.

Although it would be really nice for our periods to just stop, it doesn't always happen that way. Irregular periods, including skipped periods, heavier bleeding, longer periods, or periods coming twice a month, are common before menopause. Not every woman will have these symptoms, and those who do may not have them in severe forms. For many women, the transition to the final period is a peaceful, calm, and natural one, and one that passes quickly and without major disruption in their lives. An estimated 15–20 percent of women do not have any hot flashes at all when they go through menopause. At the other end of the spectrum, an estimated 10–20 percent of women experience severe menopausal symptoms.[1] On average, symptoms last about four years. Unfortunately, there's no way to predict where you'll fall in this spectrum. Since these symptoms are subjective, only you can determine how bothersome, if at all, they are, and whether or not you prefer to intervene in treating these symptoms.

HORMONE REPLACEMENT THERAPY

During menopause, some women suffer debilitating hot flashes or other symptoms that make their lives miserable. Hormone replacement therapy (HRT) works wonders for these symptoms, but at a potentially high price that makes this treatment a hot-button topic. In 2002, the Women's Health Initiative (WHI) released the first in a series of reports revealing that women who took combination HRT (therapy containing both estrogen and progestin) increased their risk of breast cancer. The same report also linked HRT with increased risks of heart attack, stroke, gallbladder disease, and possibly lung and even ovarian cancer. Since then, several follow-up reports have supported the initial findings in terms of the increased risk of breast cancer in particular.

In an attempt to boil down these complicated studies, the media (and even some physicians) summed everything up in a single line: HRT = breast cancer.

As usual, it's not that simple.

First, the media rarely mention a key factor: The average age of the women in the WHI patient group was sixty-three. An older age group has, by definition, a higher-than-average risk of heart attacks, strokes, and cancers. Overall, many scientists and physicians believe there were many flaws in the WHI study design, which could also skew the data.

Second, it's important to remember that we're talking about *relative* risk. Yes, women who took combination HRT had a higher risk of developing breast cancer. But in reality, HRT increased the *absolute* risk of breast cancer from five women in a hundred to six women in a hundred.[2]

Similarly, in 2010, the WHI released an update for women who took combination HRT and found that they had an increased risk of more advanced breast cancers and of dying of breast cancers. What most media did *not* report was that this risk resulted in one extra death per year for every ten thousand women taking HRT.

Then, in April 2011, doctors released yet another jaw-dropping media sound bite. Research from analysis of a subset of WHI women showed that younger postmenopausal women (in their fifties) who had had a hysterectomy and therefore did not have a uterus, and who took only estrogen as HRT, actually had as much as a 23–30 percent *reduced* risk of developing breast cancer.[3] This implied that the dangerous component was the progestin part of the HRT regimen.

Clearly, the debate continues. Research is still under way. For now, each woman's risks and benefits need to be individualized. Hormone replacement therapy is simply not a black-and-white issue where breast cancer is concerned. There are definitely risks *and* clear benefits to HRT.

As usual, how you feel about that risk depends on who you are. If you ask a breast cancer specialist about hormones, he or she may tell you to avoid them like the plague. But gynecologists, who sometimes see patients literally debilitated by menopausal symptoms, may have a different view. Personally, I try to treat the whole woman, not just one body part, taking into account the individual risks versus benefits for each particular woman. Of course, I advocate exploring all the options, and minimizing the risk by giving the lowest dose of a medication or hormone for the shortest period of time. But when patients feel they can't function with the degree of symptoms they experience, I recommend exploring HRT as an option, discussing your personal risks with your doctor, and figuring out a plan to use HRT safely and effectively. Ultimately, many factors go into causing breast cancer, and hormone exposure around menopause is but one of many. For my patients who do wish to take HRT, I usually prescribe it in bioidentical transdermal patch form.

Bioidentical Hormones

The term *bioidentical* isn't as mysterious as it sounds. It simply refers to hormones that are made from plant-based compounds rather than from a synthetic source or from the urine of pregnant horses (which is where some synthetic estrogen comes from). The name is a little misleading: There is no scientific evidence that bioidenticals are, in fact, *identical* to the hormones we have circulating in our bodies. There are two types of bioidentical hormones: those that are made by a pharmaceutical company and those that are individually compounded by a pharmacist.

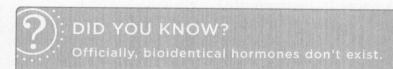

DID YOU KNOW?
Officially, bioidentical hormones don't exist.

So-called bioidentical hormones are derived from plants, not humans or animals, but there's no evidence that they're actually identical to human hormones. Both the FDA and the National Endocrine Society consider the term *bioidentical* to be nothing but marketing-speak, with no clinical, medical, or scientific meaning.

It is important to understand that having a pharmacist mix and match various plant-based hormones to your personal body type is not a treatment that has been subjected to rigorous scientific research, as other basic medical and pharmaceutical practices have. Furthermore, there is absolutely no way of knowing about the purity or composition of what you get from an individual compounding pharmacy.

While not perfect, at least prescription bioidentical hormones that come from a factory have been subjected to the standards and practices of the FDA. In addition, bioidentical formulations (either the kind made in a factory or in a compounding pharmacy) have never been studied head-to-head with synthetic hormones to assess their risk and benefit profile. I tell my patients that if they relieve symptoms and make you feel better, we have no choice at this time but to assume that they carry the same risks (or benefits) as do the higher-dose synthetic hormones.[4] That said, I use the factory-produced bioidentical form of HRT for my patients and discourage them from using unregulated individually compounded products.

Other Effects of HRT

My own mother has been on HRT in bioidentical patch form for more than twenty years. She is a healthy woman, a nonsmoker with no family history of breast cancer or heart attack. In 2002, when almost every woman in the world on HRT felt pressured to stop taking hormones, she tried to stop taking her HRT. Within two weeks, she felt physically ill. After discussing her options with her gynecologist (who's not me, by the way!), she decided to resume her HRT. She felt better in no time. The reason I share this personal anecdote with you is to illustrate how HRT can have overall systemic effects that go far beyond the hot flash. Many menopausal women experience a wide range of symptoms, including moodiness, mental dullness, body composition changes, low libido, and vaginal dryness. Treatment with HRT can alleviate many of these symptoms, although the only FDA-approved indication for HRT is the hot flash. And like any other medication or supplement, the side effects and results are variable and differ person to person. Some women feel bloated, nauseated, and even more fatigued on HRT than they did without it. Remember that whatever the reason for prescribing or taking HRT, the principle of using the lowest dose for the shortest period of time is usually the best approach.

Improving Hormone Safety

A few factors can improve the safety profile of HRT, especially regarding the risk of clotting. All hormones, including birth control pills, are associated with an increased risk of blood clots in the leg, lung, heart, and brain. But when hormones are absorbed through the skin via a patch, cream, or gel rather than ingested in pill form, the hormones bypass the liver and have less effect on clotting. Another advantage to hormones administered through the skin is that lower doses can be used, which may offset the potentially negative effects of oral hormones to a woman's cholesterol and lipid levels.

Another practice that may improve the safety of HRT involves taking the drugs cyclically—that is, taking them for several weeks, then taking a week off. A Danish study of nearly seven hundred thousand women found that women who took HRT cyclically had a lower heart attack risk than did women who took HRT continuously.[5] If you consider HRT, be sure to talk to your doctor about all of the options regarding this treatment—how to take it, when to take it, and for how long to take it. In addition, remember that being on any form of HRT (whether bioidentical or synthetic) should include follow-up appointments with your physician every six months or so, so you can be monitored for side effects and doses can be adjusted if necessary.

HERBAL THERAPIES

I'm a big believer in the power of herbs. Some of the most potent and effective medications we have and use in medicine come from plants. For this reason, I think about herbs exactly as I do prescription medications: They have benefits *and* risks. Unfortunately, lots of people forget about the risk part, assuming that herbal therapies have no side effects. The truth is, we just don't know, since most herbs haven't been studied or approved by the FDA. So I take a cautious approach to herbal treatments, and recommend that you do, too.

Herbs have gotten a lot of attention for women's hormonal complaints. Some may be safe and effective, while others may not be. Below, I'll tell you about two in particular that receive a lot of press. If you're curious about other herbal treatments, I highly recommend you check out a copy of the *Physicians' Desk Reference for Herbal Medicines*. I think it's the best resource on herbal supplements around. If you take any herbs or are considering taking any, please educate yourself (and possibly your doctor) about the possible risks and benefits of your herbal products.

Black Cohosh

Although this is a widely available herb (sometimes sold under the name Remifemin) that may alleviate menopause symptoms, I *do not* recommend this for my patients. While black cohosh seems to relieve hot flashes, some animal studies have linked it to an increased risk of breast cancer tumors that have metastasized to the lungs.[6] This makes sense. If the herb can treat symptoms caused by declining estrogen levels, it stands to reason that it may affect the breast and the uterus, because estrogen affects these organs as well. We just don't know a lot about its risks, so I can't assume it is safe for my patients.

Vitex Chasteberry

Another herb, vitex chasteberry, is used extensively in Europe as a natural treatment for a variety of hormonal conditions, from infertility to hot flashes, and is getting more and more attention in the United States. It may relieve declining progesterone effects such as bloating, fatigue, and moodiness. I have patients who report good results with vitex, although they say it can take up to twelve weeks to start to feel a difference. But again, rigorous scientific studies of vitex are still lacking. We don't know exactly how vitex works: It contains phytoestrogen (a plant form of estrogen) but may work through melatonin effects as well.[7] Studies to date have not shown significant risks with vitex, but more research is needed. Until then, with this and other herbs, please inform yourself about possible side effects, and keep yourself updated on the latest research about them

No Simple Answers

As you can see, nothing is simple when it comes to hormone imbalances or hormone replacement therapy. Here, we just scratched the surface. Every day we learn more and more about hormonal imbalances and the risks and benefits of HRT. Hopefully, in the future, bioidenticals and herbal therapies will be more thoroughly studied as well. What should be very clear by now is that the topic of hormonal imbalance should not be a two-minute discussion, where your doctor writes a prescription, hands it to you, and says "See you in a year." Talk with your doctor extensively if you think you may have an imbalance, but be sure to consider all the other, more common causes that may be contributing to your symptoms. And understand the risks and benefits of any hormonal medications or supplements you do decide to take.

Beauty and the Breast

Remember when your breasts were a big deal? Maybe you couldn't wait for them to bud, or maybe you nearly died of embarrassment wearing your first training bra. Maybe you have fond memories of your first foray into Victoria's Secret, searching for the perfect push-up bra to show them off at their beautiful best.

By the time you're in your thirties, your breasts may seem less like an intoxicating new relationship and more like a longtime marriage— the thrill may be gone, but you've been through a lot together and they've never let you down. You might even take them for granted.

As you enter your thirties and forties, though, you'll find it's time to renew your acquaintance. They need your attention, and treating them well now will help keep them beautiful and healthy in the coming decades. Most important, you need to stay abreast (sorry!) of the latest thinking in breast care, cancer prevention, and even options in breast surgery, so you can decide what's best for your breasts now and in the future. In this chapter, I'll review breast basics, but also tell you what you need to know about new developments in breast health, and new thinking about breast exams and cancer.

Who Popped the Balloons? Your Breasts Before and After Forty

Many of my patients are shocked to find their breasts changing shape as they age. They may flatten or stretch or otherwise seem to deflate. It's an age-related change that most of us don't anticipate, but it's perfectly normal.

To understand how age affects the breasts, we need to review our basic anatomy. Breasts may look like simple structures when they're filling out a bikini, but there's much more to them than meets the eye. They're made of three types of tissue: skin, fat, and glandular tissue that produces milk when the right hormones are present.

YOUR BREASTS AT THIRTY

The tissue is dense, strong, and healthy. Breasts may hurt around the time of your period, but rarely give you cause for complaint.

YOUR BREASTS AT FORTY

The tissue becomes thinner, looser, and weaker as cells separate from one another. Ligaments in the chest supporting your breasts start to weaken and they're less pert and perky as things head south. Your breasts may seem deflated, saggy, or flatter. Your nipples may get smaller and be less responsive to stimulation (either touch or temperature). Gradually, the lobules or sacs that produce milk get replaced by fat, also possibly leading to changes in breast size, shape, or feel.

YOUR BREASTS DURING PREGNANCY

If you're pregnant in your thirties or early forties, you may not see any shrinkage at all until well after pregnancy. In fact, you'll see the opposite. Breasts may grow by a cup size or more during pregnancy, and keep growing afterward. Think Kate Hudson morphing into Salma Hayek. Often, breasts are your early warning system for pregnancy, sometimes becoming sore or tender at the nipple within days of your missing a period.

During pregnancy, you may notice your breasts feel itchy, your nipples feel tender, and you may see more veins in your breasts. Your nipples may leak colostrum, or pre-milk (a thick, yellowish nipple discharge).

YOUR BREASTS AFTER
BREAST-FEEDING/PREGNANCY

Some degree of breast deflation is common as your breasts return to the status quo. But it's not true that breast-feeding ruins your breasts. Some sagging simply comes with age, so it's hard to say what's caused by breast-feeding. Like everything else involving the human body, part of the equation involves your genetics, your environment, and your behavior. There is no way to predict how your breasts will look by the time you are finished with childbearing. But the benefits of breast-feeding (see chapter 7 on pregnancy) are big enough to outweigh any slight sagging you might notice.

YOUR BREASTS IN PREMENOPAUSE

As you approach menopause, you might experience mastalgia (pain and soreness in your breasts). You might have experienced this at other times in your life, too. Although we don't really know what causes mastalgia, we do know it seems to be related to hormonal changes, possibly a response to progesterone. The pain typically affects the outer, lower portions of the breasts and is most noticeable in the two weeks before you get your period.

Try sleeping in a sports bra for added support, changing your bras altogether (nothing like a good reason to buy new bras!), reducing caffeine, and/or taking ibuprofen—400 mg every 4–6 hours—as directed on the label. All these measures can help reduce this usually temporary discomfort. If the pain gets worse or does not go away after two or three months, it's a good idea to give your doctor a call.

A Cut Above? Cosmetic Surgery for Breasts

Bigger, smaller, rounder, perkier—for at least some brief moment, we've probably all wished we could trade in our breasts. Even if you've lived in peace with your breasts for twenty years, as you age you may revisit the question, looking for a little lift to get you through the years ahead. My brother, Dr. Evan Garfein, is a plastic surgeon in New York City, and he gave me the scoop on the latest and greatest in cosmetic surgery for breasts. It's a highly individual decision and I can't tell you what's right or wrong for you. But if this is something you'd consider, I want you to know the facts. That's especially important right now, because new options are about to come on the market.

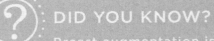

DID YOU KNOW?
Breast augmentation is the
most popular plastic surgery.

More people had breast augmentation than any other kind of plastic surgery in 2010. It beat out liposuction and eyelid surgery, the next most popular options. Breast reductions were number four on the list.[1]

PERKING UP: BREAST LIFTS

If you're bothered by sagging breasts, whether they're caused by age, dramatic weight loss, or pregnancy, a breast lift (one of the most popular cosmetic procedures for women ages thirty to thirty-nine) can improve the appearance of support and firmness, although it won't make your breasts bigger. Plastic surgeons may recommend this procedure for patients whose nipples point toward the floor or fall below the breast crease at the bottom of the breasts.

Depending on the size and shape of your breasts, the position of your nipples, the amount of sagging you have, and the quality of your skin, your surgeon will either simply cut around the areola (nipple complex), or around the areola and then vertically beneath the breast, leaving a scar that looks like a lollipop. Sometimes, breast lifts are performed in conjunction with breast reductions or breast augmentations (enlargements). The best candidates are generally healthy and don't smoke. About half of breast lifts performed are on women over forty.

BIGGER AND BETTER?
BREAST AUGMENTATION

If you've longed to fill a bikini like Angelina Jolie, you're not alone. Breast augmentation surgery is the most popular cosmetic procedure in the country, according to the American Society for Aesthetic Plastic Surgery.[2] More than a quarter of a million women have this surgery every year.

If you're thinking about breast augmentation surgery, you face a big question: Specifically, how large do you want them? Believe it or not, many plastic surgeons say the most common complaint that women have after this surgery is that their new breasts aren't big enough! On the other hand, I also have patients who feel that their ambitions were a little *too* inflated—and later had more surgery to replace their implants. As you think about the right size, remember that as you age, you'll probably put on a few pounds, some of which will go to your chest, so the result in ten years may be bigger than you planned. Last, it is important to remember that breast implants are not permanent devices, which means that if you're thirty, the odds are that you will have at least one more operation on your breasts in your lifetime. On average, implants last between ten and twenty years.

Next, you'll need to discuss the choice between saline and silicone implants with your doctor.

> Silicone implants: The FDA-approved silicone gel implants in 2006, after years of controversy about whether they increased the risk of connective tissue diseases in women. Silicone implants are generally thought to be more natural-feeling and -looking than saline implants. Manufacturers recommend that women who receive silicone implants undergo screening with an MRI every three years to check for leaks in the shell of the implants.

Saline implants: These are filled with sterile salt water. Some people feel as though these result in a more firm, less natural feel. It's easier to detect leaks in saline implants, as they simply deflate, and if a leak does occur, the salt water is simply absorbed by the body.

New implant options: Two new techniques for breast augmentations are being developed as I write this. A silicone implant known as the "gummy bear," supposedly offering a more natural feel and texture, is now in clinical trials. The second advance involves harvesting a woman's own fat cells from the abdomen or buttocks, mixing them with growth factors, and then injecting them into the breasts. The initial results are encouraging, but further research needs to be done. The most recent studies suggest that fat injections do not cause difficulties with mammography, but the impact in patients with a high risk of developing breast cancer is unknown. At this time, this procedure is not yet in clinical trials in the United States for cosmetic use, but likely will be, for both cancer reconstruction and cosmetic purposes, by 2016.

There are multiple options for where the skin will be cut. Possible incision locations include the junction between the breast and the chest wall in the fold of skin located under the breast, around the areola, or, sometimes, through a small incision in the armpit. The implant can then be placed either beneath the muscle or beneath the breast tissue and above the muscle in the breast. The best combination of implant size, shape, placement, and access incision depends on the individual patient's characteristics and the surgeon's preference. All this will be part of your discussion with your surgeon.

BREAST AUGMENTATION SURGERY RISKS

- Asymmetry: breasts might be noticeably different sizes
- Possible numbness or loss of sensation around the nipple
- Implants are not guaranteed for life and may rupture or leak
- With silicone implants, periodic MRIs may be needed to check for leaks
- If scar tissue forms due to leaks, more surgery may be needed
- Implants may interfere with breast cancer screening
- Implants may interfere with breast-feeding
- Infection
- Need for revision surgery as the patient ages and the native breast tissue changes

HONEY, I SHRUNK THE TITS: BREAST REDUCTION

While breast augmentation is usually done for cosmetic reasons, breast reduction surgery, where excess fat and skin are removed, does more than enhance a woman's appearance. Uncomfortably large breasts can create back, neck, and shoulder pain, prevent women from exercising, and produce skin irritations in addition to creating emotional distress. This procedure is especially popular among African-American women. I recommend it for any of my patients whose large breasts are creating physical or emotional discomfort. Most of my patients who have had the procedure wish they'd done it sooner.

Breast Cancer: It Could Be You

For the past few years, it's been hard to walk down a supermarket aisle without seeing a pink ribbon pop out at you from a box of oatmeal or a package of granola bars. Countless celebrities have raised their voices to promote breast cancer awareness. We've all become more aware of breast cancer. At the same time, science has become better at fighting it. While one in eight women will be diagnosed with breast cancer during her lifetime, the odds of survival are improving, and we now consider breast cancer a treatable disease.

Still, even with widespread awareness, vast confusion surrounds prevention and detection. Every month, the recommendations seem to change. Should you do breast self-exams or not? How often do you need mammograms—if at all? It's fair to say that breast cancer is the country's most widely publicized disease with the most confusing recommendations. Partly that's because this is an evolving field, with standards and practices changing as we speak. I'll clarify the facts for you here.

HOW RISKY IS "RISKY"?

That commonly known one-in-eight statistic is terrifying—but it's a little misleading. Your own personal risk may be higher or lower. For a better idea of your personal risk, go to the National Cancer Institute's website at www.cancer.gov/bcrisktool/ and answer seven simple questions. These questions are part of the Gail Model of breast cancer risk, which can give you a better idea of your own personal odds. Note that this test assesses cancer risk only for women age thirty-five and older, and is designed for use by health professionals, so you should discuss what you learn with your doctor.

The questions include:

How old are you now?

How old were you when you got your first period and had your
first baby?

What is your race or ethnic background?

Has your mother, sister, or daughter had breast cancer?

How many breast biopsies have you had?

How many of those showed a result called atypical hyperplasia?

Y ou will be given a five-year risk percentage and a lifetime risk percentage of developing breast cancer. This still isn't your own individual result—it's the risk for a group of women with similar risk
factors. Even if you're in a low-risk group, you can still get breast cancer
(just as you can still get hurt in a car accident if you wear a seat belt).
Talk to your doctor about what your Gail Model result means.

FAMILY MATTERS

If a first-degree relative—your mother, sister, or daughter—had breast
cancer, your risk is elevated. Your doctor will want to know what type
of breast cancer your family member had, and may recommend that you
start getting mammograms ten years before your mother or other relative was diagnosed, or at the age of forty, whichever comes first.

GENE SCREENS

Only 7 percent of all breast cancer cases are hereditary. But women with
a mutation in the BRCA gene, which helps suppress tumors, face a
much higher risk of breast cancer than the general female population.

Knowing if you have this mutation might have profound effects on the way you screen for cancer or on the lifestyle you choose.

BRCA genes suppress tumors by helping to repair DNA when it gets broken or damaged. When the BRCA gene is mutated, the DNA cannot get repaired and cancer can result. Half of all BRCA mutation carriers are men, which means they can pass this mutation on to their daughters (and sons). Women with certain kinds of BRCA mutations have a 60–82 percent greater risk of developing breast cancer compared to women without the mutation. If your medical records have certain red flags, like a family history of breast cancer, your doctor may recommend genetic counseling and a blood test for the BRCA mutation. Insurance will *not* be notified of your results, so a mutation won't hurt you financially.

 ## SCREENS FOR GENES: TESTING FOR MUTATIONS

If you have any of the following risk factors in your background, your doctor may recommend a BRCA test.

- A first-degree relative with breast cancer before age fifty
- A family history of male breast cancer at any age
- A family history of ovarian cancer at any age
- Eastern European Jewish (Ashkenazi) heritage with family history of breast or ovarian cancer at any age
- A family history of breast and ovarian cancer in the same person at any age
- Two different primary breast cancers in a relative of any age
- Two or more breast cancers in the family, one occurring before age fifty
- A known BRCA mutation in the family

If you have a positive result, your doctor will help you understand your options. Some women who receive positive results choose to have their breasts and ovaries removed, which has been shown to prevent cancer and save lives. Others choose more aggressive surveillance.

Checking for Cancer: What the Heck Am I Supposed to Do?

Every year, it seems as if there's a new recommendation for breast cancer screening. Do self-exams. No, wait! Don't do them! They help detect cancer. But they don't save lives. Start mammograms at forty. No, don't start until fifty!

If you're health conscious (and I hope you are), it seems hard to fathom why you wouldn't get mammograms and do your own regular breast exams. I believe your body is your responsibility, and you need to know it intimately, so if there's a change, you can notice it and bring it to the attention of a health-care provider. Indeed, some 70 percent of breast cancers are detected by self-exam!

On the other hand, self breast exams have not been shown to save lives. Eight out of ten lumps that a woman finds turn out not to be cancer, but benign masses. Viewed in this way, self-exams lead to diagnostic tests and biopsies, pain, scarring, cost, and anxiety. For this reason, the American Cancer Society's official policy sounds a little vague. It says that self breast exams should be "an option" for all women over the age of twenty. That said, all experts agree that if you feel or notice any change in your breasts—whether it's through a formal breast exam or simply something you notice—you should notify your doctor right away.

My own philosophy is that my patients should take charge of their own health and their own bodies, so I recommend that they do their own breast exams once a month, after their period.

SELF-SERVICE: YOUR BREAST EXAM

Here are the latest recommendations for performing your own breast exam. Call your doctor if you find anything new or different, as well as anything that feels like a marble or a pea, any liquid coming from your nipple, or any changes in your skin overlying the breast.

- Perform the exam at the same time every month, ideally right after your period.
- Place your hands on your hips with some pressure, and visually inspect the overall appearance of your breasts.
- Visually inspect your breast for any skin changes or dimpling.
- Feel your whole breast while lying down, standing up, and leaning over, using light, medium, and deep pressure.
- Move your fingers up and down in a vertical pattern over the entire breast.
- Check behind the nipple and into the armpit.
- Check your armpit with your arm loosely and slightly raised overhead, not straight up or bent back.

If you would like to examine your breasts, but aren't sure how to do it, ask your doctor. There really is no wrong way to do a self breast exam!

The Latest on Mammograms

In 2009, an uproar broke out over mammogram recommendations. For years, the U.S. Preventive Services Task Force, a group of researchers making recommendations to doctors and insurance companies, recommended that women receive mammograms every year or two to screen for breast cancer starting at age forty. But in 2009, the group changed its stand and recommended that routine mammograms start at fifty, except for women with a higher-than-average risk of breast cancer.

These recommendations were met with passionate and often angry reactions. I spoke on *CBS Evening News* with Katie Couric and CBS's *Face the Nation* with Bob Schieffer about these recommendations, noting that while mammography is the best screening imaging test we have to detect breast cancer, it's a long way from perfect, especially for women in their forties. In a nutshell, the recommendations changed because the task force found that mammograms weren't shown to prevent as many deaths for women in their forties as they do for older women—and they created risks and problems that some people felt outweighed benefits. (Of course, other studies found that mammograms do save lives even for younger women.)

Mammograms yield many false positives (results that show something abnormal that turns out not to be cancer) and there are even false negatives (a "normal" result when cancer is actually present). This leads to unnecessary tests and biopsies, which have their own risks, and may create anxiety. Mammograms also expose women to a small amount of radiation. Still, as of 2010, the American Cancer Society and the American College of Obstetricians and Gynecologists continues to recommend yearly mammograms for all women starting at age forty, and younger if they are at high risk, and I agree with these guidelines. My feeling is that, until we have something better, women in their forties should continue to have the option to receive mammograms, as long as they understand the limitations of the test and the risks involved.

JUST THE FACTS, MAMM(OGRAMS)

- You can still have a mammogram if you are breast-feeding.
- You can still have a mammogram if you have implants.
- A mammogram can find cancer approximately two years before it would be felt by a woman or her doctor.
- Mammograms sometimes yield false positives or false negatives, so they're not perfect by a long shot.

In 2011, some doctors began using a new kind of mammogram based on 3-D imagery, which may be more accurate than conventional mammograms. Research suggests the 3-D mammogram increases a doctor's ability to spot cancer by 7 percent and decreases false positives. Though this new 3-D mammogram does use slightly more radiation than conventional mammograms, many radiologists feel it will eventually replace the 2-D technology. Researchers are evaluating the new approach to see if it actually saves more lives. If you're considering a mammogram, ask your doctor, your breast imaging center, and your insurance company to see if this newer technology is available and appropriate for you, and what it might cost.

WHAT IF I CAN'T AFFORD A MAMMOGRAM?

On average, mammograms cost several hundred dollars—a painful wallop if you don't have insurance. Fortunately, there are ways to get a mammogram for less, or even for free if you don't have insurance. Some cities have mobile buses that travel around offering mammograms to women without insurance. Many hospitals have free breast screening clinics. And last, some private radiology centers will negotiate sliding fees for mammograms for women without insurance. So before you assume you can't afford one, ask imaging centers and health-care providers about lower cost options.

DID YOU KNOW?

There is frequently discrimination in reconstructive surgery.

When discussing surgery for breast cancer, a woman with health insurance is more likely to be offered reconstruction than a woman without insurance. Sad but true. However, things are changing. Several states are requiring hospitals and doctors to discuss all reconstructive options with their patients prior to mastectomy, regardless of whether or not they have health insurance. In New York state, my brother was instrumental in convincing former governor David Paterson to pass a law to this effect.

Other Breast Tests

While mammograms are the most widely used tool for detecting breast cancer, some doctors have started using other screening tests as well.

SONOGRAMS

Sonograms, or ultrasounds (the terms are interchangeable), are often done along with mammography to evaluate breast tissue for women in their thirties and forties. Ultrasounds use sound waves, not radiation, to look at structures within the breast. They show whether a lump is solid or cystic (fluid-filled). In some women with dense breasts or cystic breasts, or who are at high risk for breast cancer, ultrasounds are routinely ordered along with mammograms. I recommend my patients stagger these tests, scheduling one at the beginning of the year and one six months later. It may be less convenient than scheduling them at the same time, but this ensures that no more than half a year goes by without some type of breast imaging, which is important for women with a high cancer risk.

MAGNETIC RESONANCE IMAGING

Magnetic resonance imaging (MRI) uses magnetic waves, instead of sound waves (like sonograms) or X-rays (like mammograms), to evaluate the breasts. Often, an intravenous dye or contrast material is administered through an IV to make the images easier to read. MRIs are actually better than mammograms at detecting cancers, but they also give more false positives. For this reason, MRIs are only recommended for women with high breast cancer risk as a supplement to mammograms, and not recommended for women at average risk for breast cancer.

Note that breast MRIs require different equipment than an MRI of the head or pelvis. Not all imaging facilities have the special equipment needed for breast MRIs, so be sure to ask the facility if it has the ability to perform MRI-guided breast biopsies. Otherwise, if it turns out you need a biopsy, you'd have to have the MRI repeated at another facility where the biopsy could be performed.[3]

Preventing Breast Cancer

Many factors that increase your breast cancer risk are completely out of your control. After all, you had no say in when you got your period, or what your race or ethnic background is. The good news is, several critical factors *are* under your control. By limiting alcohol, losing weight, and exercising, you can reduce the risk of developing breast cancer. These recommendations are probably familiar, because they prevent other diseases, too.

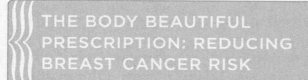

THE BODY BEAUTIFUL PRESCRIPTION: REDUCING BREAST CANCER RISK

To reduce your risk of breast cancer, develop the following lifetime habits. (By the way, it's no coincidence that many of these are promoted already in the Body Beautiful prescriptions for diet, fitness, etc., so if you build those habits you'll reduce your breast cancer risk automatically!)

- Limit alcohol to seven or fewer drinks a week.
- Lose weight if you are overweight or obese.
- Exercise (some is better than none, more is better than less).
- Take 1,000 IU of vitamin D_3 daily.
- If possible, breast-feed your babies.
- Discuss your personal risks versus benefits regarding hormone replacement therapy with your doctor.

LIMIT ALCOHOL

According to the National Cancer Institute, alcohol increases the risk of breast cancer. The more alcohol you drink, the greater your risk. Even moderate consumption (defined as about one drink per day, or seven drinks a week) increases cancer risk. Specifically, women who have one or more drinks a day face twice the risk of a type of cancer called lobular carcinoma (which represents about 10–15 percent of all breast cancers) than women who drink less. However, alcohol does not seem to increase the risk for ductal-type breast cancer, which accounts for 70 percent of cases.[4]

LOSE WEIGHT

You hear this over and over, like an iPod stuck on repeat, but people at a healthy weight have lower risks for all kinds of diseases, including cancer. If you are overweight or obese, lose weight *now*, in your thirties and forties, before menopause. One study found that women who lost weight from the age of thirty until menopause reduced their risk of getting breast cancer.[5] If you're already at a healthy weight, work hard to stay there; maintaining a healthy weight also lowered risk.

Even if you don't need to lose weight, eating a healthy, low-fat diet may reduce your risk of developing breast cancer, or of reducing your risk of recurrence. In one study, women with breast cancer who reduced fat to approximately 15 percent of their total daily caloric intake had a 24–42 percent reduction in the risk of cancer recurrence, compared to women whose fat intake was 30 percent of their total daily calories.[6]

GET MOVING

You probably knew that exercise reduces breast cancer risk. But did you know that even the exercise you did way back in high school may still be working to protect your breasts? Another great reason to encourage our daughters to play sports!

But even if you didn't start young, it's never too late to reap the benefits of exercise. One study found that brisk walking for as little as one hour and fifteen minutes a week reduced the cancer risk by 18 percent![7] That's only about eleven minutes a day! Other studies, however, suggest that more strenuous exercise is needed.

If possible, exercise for forty-five to sixty minutes almost every day.

I know it sounds impossible, but think of the rewards (and see chapter 2 for advice on getting started).

VITAMIN D$_3$

If you read chapter 1, you already know about recent research showing that vitamin D$_3$ supplements may help with all kinds of diseases and conditions, from heart disease to depression. Now we also know that this fat-soluble vitamin (found in sunlight, some fortified foods like milk, eggs, and salmon, and in supplements) may reduce your breast cancer risk. One study found that premenopausal women with the highest dietary and supplemental intakes of vitamin D$_3$ and calcium had at least a 30 percent reduction in their risk of breast cancer.[8] Research has also shown that women with early breast cancer who have low levels of vitamin D have a higher risk of recurrence and death, and women with low levels of vitamin D are also at higher risk of developing breast cancer in the first place.[9]

It's important to remember that these and other such studies regarding vitamin D and cancer generally show an association between the two, rather than a cause-and-effect explanation. In other words, we don't really know exactly how they're related. More research is happening now. In the meantime, it's a good idea to take a vitamin D$_3$ supplement every day. You don't need to take much to make a difference. One study found that women who got approximately 550 IU of vitamin D$_3$ a day had a 35 percent lower risk of breast cancer than those women who got the least vitamin D. The protective effect was seen most dramatically in women with the more aggressive types of tumors, which often affect younger women.[10]

Remember that too much of a good thing can be a *bad* thing; vitamin D is no exception. The Institute of Medicine recommends no more than 4,000 IU of vitamin D$_3$ a day. More than that can cause kidney stones (ouch!) and other problems. Make sure you talk to your doctor about using a vitamin D_3 supplement.

BREAST-FEED

You already know that breast-feeding is good for your baby, but it's also good for you. Numerous studies have demonstrated that breast-feeding is associated with a reduced risk of breast cancer. (It's also linked to lower risks of ovarian cancer, osteoporosis, hypertension, and heart disease.) The theory goes like this: Lactation suppresses ovulation, which means there's less hormonal stimulation to your body, including your breasts, during the time when you're lactating—and anything that reduces the hormonal stimulation of the breast can be protective against cancer. One recent study, which used data from the large and reputable Harvard Nurses' Health Study, found that for women who breast-fed and who also had a first-degree relative with breast cancer, the risk of getting pre-menopausal breast cancer was 59 percent less than women who had a first-degree relative with breast cancer but did not breast-feed.[11] It's not yet clear, however, how long a woman should breast-feed to get the maximal benefits, but for now, any breast-feeding is better than none.

Breast Cancer Today

If you or someone you love is diagnosed with breast cancer, remember that things are very different today from even a decade or two ago. Breast cancer survivors are everywhere, and you have a wide variety of treatment options. In fact, emerging evidence suggests that not all breast cancer actually needs aggressive treatment, and that some breast cancers will never go on to cause death. Of course, no one likes the idea of living with cancer cells in her body, but the big message is: Take your time.

First, get a second or even a third opinion. Then, take your time in deciding about treatments. Speak to several doctors about the options of lumpectomy versus mastectomy with or without reconstruction. Understand that many options regarding reconstruction are affected by the initial treatment, so try to think into the future about reconstruction even before you begin initial treatment. You may feel that you need to rush through treatment decisions, but the reality is, you don't. Typically, you have plenty of time to collect all the information you need and think about your options. Being informed about your treatment options, your prognosis, and about your own breasts, even when they're healthy, is the best thing you can do to protect yourself from cancer, now and in the future.

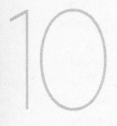

The Heart of the Matter

Keeping Your Ticker Ticking

et's cut right to the chase: An estimated one in three women has heart disease. One in three. That means you're more likely to have heart disease than to have blue eyes (one in six),[1] graduate from college (about one in four),[2] or speak a foreign language (one in four).[3] You're also more likely to die from heart disease than from *anything else*.

Heart disease is the number-one killer of women.

That means you, personally, are very likely to die of heart disease.

And yet *not a single one* of my patients thinks these statistics apply to her. We all think we're the exception. We tell ourselves because we exercise, we eat right, no one in our family had heart disease, or we're too young, the odds don't apply to us. Nationally, only 13 percent of women admit that heart disease is the greatest threat to their own health, and less than half recognize that heart disease is such a big killer, despite a long, intense campaign by the American Heart Association.[4] It's sort of reverse sexism. No matter how many times we hear otherwise, we think heart disease and heart attacks are something for men to worry about, not women.

For an eye-opener, take the quick quiz below.

HEART HEALTH: TRUE OR FALSE?

- Women are more likely to die after a heart attack than men.
- Death rates due to heart disease in women ages thirty-five to fifty-four are rising.
- One in three adults has hypertension.

These are all true. Surprised? Motivated? Keep reading to learn how you can lower your risks.

Your Personal Risk

If you've read this far into the book, you know that the key to keeping your body beautiful is staying healthy and strong. You need to understand your personal risks and how to reduce them to live a long, healthy, energetic life. Fortunately, the measures that prevent heart disease also help you look and feel younger, more vibrant, and more energetic. The side effects of preventing heart disease would be worth it even if they didn't help your heart!

In this chapter, I'll quickly lay out the basic healthy habits you need to develop to prevent heart disease. No surprises here. You're probably already working on some of them through the Body Beautiful prescriptions. Later in the chapter, I'll give you a careful breakdown of several kinds of heart diseases, risk factors, and how you can assess and manage your own risk.

? **WHAT'S YOUR RISK OF HEART DISEASE?**

The American Heart Association offers an online risk calculator that can help to assess your own risk over the next ten years. (Go to www.heart .org and search for "heart attack risk assessment.")

THE BODY BEAUTIFUL PRESCRIPTION: HEART HEALTHY HABITS

Every disease has risk factors that increase your odds of getting it. Some of those odds, like family history, are beyond your control. But with heart disease, many risk factors relate to your lifestyle and can be reduced by healthy habits. By developing these habits in your thirties and forties, you can keep your heart younger, strong, and healthy in the decades ahead.

1. **If you smoke, stop immediately.** This is the single most important thing you can do for your health, and for the health of those around you. Every kind of smoking is bad for you—firsthand, secondhand (the smoke from another person's cigarettes), and thirdhand (the solid, particulate matter that settles on your hair, clothes, and furniture—not only does it stink, it's dangerous). If you think you're fine because you "only smoke at bars" or "only in the car," thirdhand smoke dangers mean you're putting others at risk as well as yourself.

   If you smoke, use every tool at your disposal to quit. Nicotine replacement therapy (sold in patch or gum form), prescription medications, hypnosis, and behavioral therapy can all be effective. Make a plan, tell everyone you know about your goal (social support is key), set a date, anticipate obstacles, and do it. Now.

2. **Exercise.** We've already talked a lot about the benefits of exercise. If you haven't started a new, or more vigorous, program already, go back and read chapter 2 again! Even though we all know how important it is to be active, only 30 percent of women in the United States get regular, strenuous exercise. The American Heart Association says you need at least two and a half hours of moderate exercise or seventy-five minutes a week of strenuous exercise (or some combination of the two) for heart health. Following the recommendations in chapter 2 (weight training at least twice a week, and interval training four times a week for at least twenty minutes) will help you reach maximum heart health.

I know it's hard to find time, but you need to make this a priority. Recruit a friend, spouse, or pet and make this part of your daily routine. The more you exercise, the more your body's natural feel-good chemicals will be produced, giving you the natural high that so many fitness addicts enjoy. And you'll look beautiful and keep a healthy weight as a side benefit.

3. **Eat a heart-healthy diet.** A diet high in fresh fruits and vegetables, fiber, whole grains (like brown rice, whole-wheat breads, and pasta), and oil-rich fish like salmon has been shown to be protective against heart disease. On the flip side, foods high in saturated fat, trans-fat, sodium, and sugar will hurt your heart health.

Read the labels and the nutritional facts on packages of food before you buy the item. For advice on healthy eating, see chapter 1.

4. **Limit salt.** When you eat salt, your body retains water to balance the sodium. For people with healthy hearts and kidneys, this usually presents no problem. But for people with heart disease or high blood pressure, this can be dangerous. The new daily re-

commended maximum salt intake is no more than 1,500 mg a day. This corresponds to approximately half a teaspoon of salt a day. It sounds like it should be easy to do, but salt hides in foods that may surprise you, like cereal. Restaurant meals often include too much salt, so limit it by asking for dressings and sauces on the side.

5. **Eat omega-3 fatty acids.** Studies have shown that consumption of omega-3 fatty acids reduces the risk of heart disease and of death from all causes. Whether you get omega-3 fatty acids from eating oily fish, such as salmon, or in supplement form, the American Heart Association recommends that women should get 500–1,800 mg a day of the EPA and DHA types of omega-3 fatty acids, or eat at least two servings a week of salmon or other oily fish. This may be particularly important for women with high cholesterol or high triglycerides. As I mentioned in chapter 1, I recommend an omega-3 fatty acid supplement daily.

6. **Lose weight.** Being even slightly overweight can increase your risk of heart disease. Sometimes losing just 5 percent of your total body weight is enough to make a big difference in preventing heart disease (so, for instance, if you weigh 170 pounds, losing just 8.5 pounds will make you healthier). Another helpful guideline is your body mass index (BMI). Your risk of heart disease is lower if your BMI is less than 25. Your risk of heart disease is also lower if your waist measures less than 35 inches. For advice on reaching these goals, revisit chapters 1 and 2.

7. **Control blood pressure and cholesterol.** For a healthy heart, you need blood pressure at or below 120/80. You also need healthy cholesterol levels. Cholesterol refers to a set of numbers called your lipid panel. It includes LDL (bad cholesterol—think L for *lousy*), HDL (good cholesterol—remember H for *healthy*), your total cholesterol, and your triglycerides. Cholesterol is not all bad; in fact, our cells need cholesterol to function well, and we need

cholesterol to produce our body's hormones. But, like anything, there's a limit. Your "lousy" cholesterol, LDL, should be less than 100, and your "healthy" cholesterol, HDL, should be over 46. Finally, your triglycerides, which are other important lipids in your body, should be less than 150.

8. **An aspirin a day?** For women at high risk for heart disease, taking an aspirin a day is usually recommended. Research shows that aspirin can reduce inflammation associated with heart disease and inhibit the formation of blood clots. But discuss risks with your doctor first, since aspirin can cause internal bleeding and stomach upset.

? WHAT DO THOSE BLOOD PRESSURE NUMBERS MEAN?

The top number of your blood pressure is called the systolic pressure, and it measures the amount of pressure that your blood exerts against your arteries when your heart beats. That number should be less than or equal to 120.

The bottom number is the diastolic pressure, and it measures the force on your arteries between heartbeats. This number should be less than or equal to 80. Overall, you want your blood pressure to be less than or equal to 120/80.

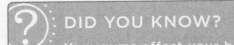

DID YOU KNOW?

Your gums affect your heart.

Having gum disease or badly decayed teeth can increase your risk of heart disease. The theory is that inflammation in the gums may cause bacteria from the mouth to travel throughout the body, attaching to fatty substances in the blood and lodging in the arteries that supply the heart with blood. See your dentist regularly for cleanings to ensure healthy gums *and* a healthy heart.[5]

Working on the factors above will lower your risk for heart disease—and may or may not lower your blood pressure and cholesterol, too. I encourage my patients to make lifestyle changes first, and if after three to six months their blood pressure and cholesterol haven't fallen to healthy levels, to try medication. If your doctor starts you on medications, you'll need close follow-up to make sure that your numbers reach a normal range and you don't suffer from side effects.

DID YOU KNOW?

Depression and heart disease are linked.

Likely due to a combination of biological and behavioral factors, women with depression are more likely to suffer a heart attack and to die of heart disease. If you have symptoms of depression, get treatment. For advice on mood management, see chapter 4.

Matters of the Heart: Defining Heart Disease

One reason heart disease affects so many women is that the term *heart disease* includes several different types of disease, all of which can be deadly. Here's a quick description of each, in order of how common they are. Fortunately, the habits I outlined in the last section will lower your risk for all of these.

CORONARY ARTERY DISEASE (CAD), OR ISCHEMIC HEART DISEASE

Quick Facts
- Clogged arteries send less oxygenated blood to the heart.
- This is the most common type of heart disease in women.
- 240,000 women die of this disease every year in the United States.
- CAD is more common in women after menopause.

What Is It?
Coronary artery disease affects the arteries that supply blood to the heart muscle. Think of these arteries as water pipes. As pipes age, corrosion and sediment can slowly block the conduit, essentially narrowing the pipe from inside. With coronary artery disease, plaques (buildups of hardened fat and other substances) clog the arteries, so less oxygenated blood makes it to the heart. During exercise or stress, this narrowing in the blood vessel means the heart may not get the extra oxygen it

needs. If a plaque suddenly detaches from the artery wall, it can cause a sudden blockage of blood and cause a heart attack.

Causes

A variety of factors can lead to CAD, including family history, high cholesterol, diabetes, and obesity. Sometimes CAD can develop in someone who has *none* of these risk factors. Another theory as to why plaques develop has to do with inflammation. There is some evidence that chronic inflammation causes blood cells and fat substances to adhere to the insides of blood vessels. This is why we say that there is a connection between poor dental health and heart disease. Gum disease can lead to microscopic amounts of bacteria circulating through the bloodstream, which causes chronic inflammation throughout the body, especially in the blood vessels that supply the heart.

Symptoms

You may have no symptoms at all while CAD is developing, or you may notice a feeling of pressure, tightness, or pain in the chest while exercising, called angina.

Risk Factors

- Family history of heart disease
- Diabetes
- High blood pressure
- High cholesterol or high triglycerides
- Obesity
- Smoking
- Age (women are more likely to develop this after menopause than before)
- Inactive lifestyle

Treatment

Treatments for CAD are usually specialized to the individual patient, but there are some general principles.

- **Control cholesterol:** The easy way to remember how to decipher these numbers is that you want your "lousy" cholesterol (LDL) to be under 100, and your "healthy" cholesterol (HDL) to be as high as possible but definitely greater than 46. Women with CAD need to do this via lifestyle *and* medication.
- **Control diabetes:** Women with diabetes need to control their blood sugar levels. Sometimes more than one medication is needed.
- **Control high blood pressure:** Since uncontrolled blood pressure is a cause of CAD, maintaining your blood pressure in the healthy range is important for women with CAD. There are many types of blood pressure medication; making sure you are on the right one, at the dose that works, is critical. Usually, women who have CAD are placed on a type called a beta-blocker.
- **Good nutrition and exercise:** Speak with your cardiologist about developing a diet and exercise program that's right for you.

HYPERTENSIVE HEART DISEASE, OR HIGH BLOOD PRESSURE

Quick Facts

- Hypertension doesn't mean you're hyper or tense. It means your blood moves through your arteries with more force and pressure, which can damage arteries over time.
- One in three adults in the United States has hypertension.
- Only about 60 percent of women with hypertension receive treatment.[6]

- Even when women do receive treatment, many (about 30 percent) do not reach blood pressure levels associated with lower risk (blood pressure less than 140/80).

What Is It?

Hypertension, or high blood pressure, forces the heart to work harder to pump blood with each heartbeat. It's like trying to open a car door against a strong wind (or, more accurately, against water, if your car were parked in a river). The wind or water (or, in your heart's case, the blood) generate so much pressure that it's much harder to open the door (or the heart valve). As a result, your heart works harder.

The hard work causes the main pumping chamber of the heart (the left ventricle) to become abnormally thickened and enlarged, making it less efficient at pumping blood to the rest of the body. Because it's less efficient, it has to work harder to do the same amount of work. Meanwhile, more and more collagen is deposited within the heart muscle as a response to this increased workload, making it stiffer and less able to open fully, preventing blood from entirely filling the chamber on each beat. Within the arteries supplying the heart muscle itself, resistance can build up (think of it as drinking a smoothie through a cocktail straw) making it more difficult for oxygen-rich blood to feed the heart muscle, which leads to a condition known as coronary insufficiency. Any of these negative consequences can cause the heart and kidneys to fail.

Causes

Often the cause is unknown, but sometimes these factors lead to hypertension:

- Medications (birth control pills, stimulants)
- Stress

- Obesity
- Smoking
- Problems with the arteries that lead to the kidneys

Symptoms

Hypertension is sometimes called the silent killer because it often produces no symptoms at all. When it does produce symptoms, you might have dizziness, headaches, blurry vision, chest pain, or shortness of breath.

Risk Factors

As for many cardiovascular diseases, the risk factors include obesity, smoking, family history, and age.

Treatment

- Lifestyle changes (less salt, healthier diet, exercise, weight loss)
- Prescription medications, including diuretics (aka water pills) and other blood pressure medications

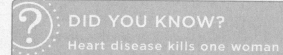

DID YOU KNOW?
Heart disease kills one woman every minute.

Heart disease causes approximately one death per minute among women in the United States.[7]

VALVULAR HEART DISEASE

Quick Facts

- Valvular conditions include heart murmurs, like the very common mitral valve prolapse.
- Heart valve problems often affect younger women.
- Eight out of a hundred women have some degree of aortic regurgitation (a valve problem described below).
- Weight-loss drugs containing fenfluramine and dexfenfluramine, aka fen-phen, are associated with increased risk of heart valve problems.
- All heart valve problems can be managed with medication and/or surgery, depending on the severity of the symptoms.

What Is It?

Your heart has four valves: The tricuspid and the pulmonic on the right, and the mitral and the aortic on the left. They're like automatic doors at a grocery store, automatically opening and closing. For women of child-bearing age, the ones on the left—the aortic and mitral valves—are the most commonly affected.

Aortic Valve Problems

Blood passes through the aortic valve as it moves from the left ventricle into the aorta (the body's main artery). Sometimes this valve doesn't close completely—it's floppy—and some blood regurgitates, or washes back into the heart instead of moving into the rest of the body. This back-wash is called aortic insufficiency (AI). If the regurgitation is severe, or in situations like pregnancy that stress the cardiovascular system, blood can eventually back up into the lungs, causing respiratory problems. Also, if severe, not enough blood will be ejected in a forward direction from the heart, causing the rest of the body to receive less blood and oxygen.[8]

Symptoms

If mild, no symptoms may be present. More severe cases can cause palpitations, chest pain, and shortness of breath.

Risk Factors

Women with lupus, Marfan syndrome, other connective tissue disorders, or who were born with a condition called bicuspid aortic valve have a higher risk of AI.

Treatment

Aortic valve problems can be managed with medications if not severe, or with surgery if necessary.

Mitral Valve Prolapse

The mitral valve sits on the left side of the heart between the upper and lower chambers. Mitral valve prolapse (MVP) happens when the valve becomes floppy and permits regurgitation, just like the aortic valve problem described above. The most common valve problem for women, MVP affects six out of a hundred women and is commonly diagnosed in young women, even teenagers. Usually, MVP is not dangerous and does not cause any significant symptoms. If severe, it can cause the same blood flow issues as severe aortic insufficiency.[9]

Symptoms

- Palpitations
- Fatigue

- Anxiety
- Chest pain
- 60 percent of patients with MVP have no symptoms at all.

RISK FACTORS
There are no standard risk factors for MVP. It can affect anyone.

TREATMENT
In the past, it was recommended that women with any degree of MVP take antibiotics before dental and other procedures to reduce the risk of infection of the valve leaflets with bacteria "liberated" during the course of these procedures. Now the recommendations have changed and only patients who have artificial heart valves or who have had endocarditis before should take antibiotics preventively.

Mitral Valve Stenosis
With this condition, the mitral valve sticks and doesn't let enough blood through.

SYMPTOMS
The symptoms can take decades to develop, but when severe they include shortness of breath, fatigue, palpitations, and coughing up pink-tinged sputum.

RISK FACTORS
Mitral valve stenosis is often caused by childhood rheumatic fever, so it's common among women who immigrated from other countries.

TREATMENT
Managed with medication or surgery. Pregnant women with mitral valve stenosis are followed closely for signs that the blood flow is back-

ing up into the lungs. Their OBs try to manage labor to avoid fluid overload and strenuous pushing during delivery.

STRESS CARDIOMYOPATHY, OR POOR HEART MUSCLE FUNCTION

What Is It?

In cardiomyopathy, a weakened heart muscle cannot pump blood effectively.

Causes

If you've ever watched a soap opera where someone fainted or had a heart attack on learning that the hero's stepsister's brother's lover was dead . . . that *could* actually happen, although it's extremely uncommon. On rare occasions, sudden and extreme emotional stress—the sudden death of a close friend or relative, or a brush with death in a car accident—has led to cardiomyopathy. These cases, which have largely occurred in women, often mimic the signs and symptoms of a heart attack, with abnormal EKG and echocardiogram readings as well as elevated blood enzyme tests for heart muscle injury. The theory is that extreme distress triggers the blood to produce chemicals called catecholamines to attack the heart in a type of toxic reaction. While this is rare, it does lend credibility to the idea that you can nearly die of a broken heart.

Symptoms

- Shortness of breath
- Swelling of the extremities

- Dizziness
- Fatigue
- Chest pain

Risk Factors
It appears that women are more at risk for stress cardiomyopathy than men.

Treatment
Treatments are the same as for other forms of cardiomyopathy and include aggressive medication in a hospital setting.

POSTPARTUM CARDIOMYOPATHY
What Is It?
Postpartum cardiomyopathy is poor heart function of a mother after giving birth. This condition can be life-threatening, with a risk of death as high as 50 percent. Because this is such a critical and dangerous condition, it is important that doctors make the correct diagnosis as quickly as possible. Unfortunately, historically this does not happen. Some studies show that more than a week goes by before postpartum cardiomyopathy is diagnosed in over 48 percent of women.[10]

Symptoms
- Shortness of breath
- Rapid heart rate
- Rapid respiratory rate
- Extreme swelling of the legs (which can be common in pregnancy)
- Cough

- Low blood oxygen level
- Difficulty breathing when lying flat
- Chest pain

Risk Factors

Mothers who have just given birth are at risk. This condition affects one in thirteen hundred to fifteen thousand women delivering babies each year.[11] Forty-five percent of cases occur in the first week following delivery, and 75 percent occur in the first month postpartum.

Treatment

Women with these symptoms should be immediately evaluated in a hospital setting and should undergo extensive testing, including blood tests, EKGs, chest X-rays, and echocardiograms. Though we still don't know exactly what causes postpartum cardiomyopathy, we do know how to treat it. Women whose heart function recovers need to be followed closely by cardiologists who specialize in heart failure. They should also avoid pregnancy in the future. When the heart muscle does not recover, a heart transplant may be required.

? DID YOU KNOW?

If you had a heart defect corrected, you may still be at risk.

There are over forty thousand babies with congenital heart defects born in the United States each year. Some of these are detected in utero with obstetric ultrasounds and are corrected with surgery soon after birth. As a result, there are many adults in the United States who have had their heart defects corrected. This can include numerous conditions such as atrial septal defect (ASD, aka a hole in the heart), Tetralogy of Fallot, and Ebstein's anomaly. If you were born with a heart defect, it is a good idea to be followed by a cardiologist who specializes in adult congenital heart disease.

SYNDROME X: SYMPTOMS IN SEARCH OF A DISEASE

A mysterious condition called syndrome X is more common in women than men. Patients experience tightness, pain, or pressure in their chests, either at rest or with exercise, but have no problems with their arteries. Previously, some experts suspected an estrogen deficiency caused this, but now doctors believe this may represent a microscopic abnormality in the blood vessels. Some studies have found that women with syndrome X and with abnormal functioning of the inner lining of their heart's blood vessels have a 30 percent chance of developing heart disease within ten years.[12]

Know Your Symptoms

You probably see a pattern: Many forms of heart disease have similar symptoms, which only makes sense, since these conditions all affect the heart. The most important thing to understand is that when you have certain symptoms of heart disease or, worse, a heart attack, it's critical for you to recognize them and respond.

You will notice that these symptoms can also be caused by other conditions, such as allergies, overconsumption of caffeine, anxiety, depression, or lung problems. You don't have to figure out what's causing them—your job is to notice them and tell your health-care provider.

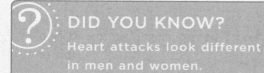

DID YOU KNOW?
Heart attacks look different
in men and women.

It's very important to know that the symptoms of a heart attack are very different for women than they are for men. Because of this, doctors as well as patients may not initially suspect a heart attack in a woman. Unexplained fatigue, weakness, and shortness of breath are the most common symptoms in women (whereas chest pain is the most common symptom in men). Knowing this difference could save your life!

Heart Attack Symptoms: Call 9-1-1

If you feel these symptoms and think you may be having a heart attack, chew an aspirin immediately (unless you're allergic) and *call 911*. Getting immediate emergency medical attention is key, since time wasted equals heart muscle lost.

- Chest pain, pressure, or tightness
- Unexplained fatigue (experienced by 43 percent of women having heart attacks)
- Weakness (experienced by 54 percent of women having heart attacks)

- Disturbed sleep
- Shortness of breath (approximately 58 percent of women having heart attacks)
- Nausea
- Sweating
- Dizziness
- Back pain
- Abdominal discomfort that feels like indigestion

Heart Disease Symptoms: Talk to Your Doctor ASAP

- Palpitations
- Leg swelling
- Poor exercise tolerance
- Awakening at night with breathing difficulties

PREGNANCY AND YOUR HEART

Pregnancy places your heart and vascular system under extreme stress. Early in pregnancy, your circulating blood volume increases by 50 percent, and by the end of the pregnancy, your heart is pumping blood not just to sustain one living person, but two (sometimes more). Problems you might think of as strictly pregnancy- or ob-gyn-related can affect your heart health later, so your primary-care physician needs to know about them. Specifically, preeclampsia (high blood pressure during pregnancy) can increase your risk of future heart disease. One study found that women with preeclampsia faced twice the risk for future heart disease and stroke in the five to fifteen years following their pregnancies.[13] Likewise, if you had gestational diabetes, you have a higher risk of developing type 2 diabetes in the future, which increases your risk of heart disease.

? DID YOU KNOW?
Metabolic syndrome increases heart risk.

Some women with a common hormonal imbalance called polycystic ovarian syndrome (PCOS) may be at higher risk for heart attack and stroke. That's because these women may also have metabolic syndrome, a collection of symptoms including high blood pressure, insulin resistance or prediabetes, high cholesterol or triglycerides, and abdominal obesity. All these, as well as an increased clotting risk, put women with metabolic syndrome at higher risk for heart attack and stroke.

Last but Not Least: Partner with Your Doctor

Knowing your own body and recognizing potential problems is your responsibility: You are your own best health advocate. But your doctor is your best partner in protecting your health. So the final, critically important factor in preventing heart disease is making sure your doctor knows all she or he needs to about your heart health.

Know Your History

The more you know about your health history, the better. Ask yourself the following questions and be sure to share the answers with your doctor, even if he or she forgets to ask. Most important, make sure you know as much as possible about your family's heart health history (especially your parents or siblings). If your parents are alive, it's a good idea to ask them for copies of their medical records so that you can pass these along to your doctor.

- Did anyone in your family die for any reason under the age of fifty?
- Is there a history of sudden death during sleep, exercise, or emotional stress in your family?
- Did anyone in your family ever have a heart attack? At what age?
- Is there anyone in your family with a pacemaker? How old and why?
- Do you smoke, drink alcohol, or use any recreational drugs? If you use or used drugs, what kinds, for how long, and how much?
- Do you exercise? What kinds of exercise do you do?
- Do you have diabetes, high cholesterol, high blood pressure, or high triglycerides?
- Do you have a waist measurement greater than 35 inches?
- Do you take any medications, herbs, or supplements?
- Have you ever had preeclampsia or diabetes during pregnancy?

Heart Tests: What to Expect

If your doctor thinks you're at high risk for heart disease, he or she may recommend one of a seemingly endless list of tests. Studies show that some tests are more accurate for women than for men. Not every test is right for every woman; much of it depends on whether your doctor thinks you are at low, medium, or high risk for heart disease, and whether you have any symptoms. Here's a quick glossary of tests you might encounter.

EKG or ECG: The doctor will attach wires to your body via sticky patches and connect them to the EKG machine, which will record the electrical activity of your heart in less than one minute. The EKG can reveal if you're having a heart attack, if you've had past "silent" heart attacks you never knew about, and how fast, how regular, and in what rhythm your heart is beating. These machines may print out their own interpretation of your heart's activities, but the results should always be evaluated by a physician, too.

Stress Test: Two types of stress tests can assess your risk of heart disease. In the first, you walk or run on a treadmill as fast as you can for a given number of minutes while an EKG records your heart activity. Before the test, an echo or sonogram measures how your heart moves, and then is repeated immediately after peak exercise to see if the exertion resulted in any decline in your heart's muscle function. This is called a stress echo. Data have shown that this test is more accurate for women than a standard exercise EKG test.[14]

In the second type of stress test, drugs such as adenosine or dobutamine are used to affect blood flow. Nuclear materials are used in conjunction with these drugs in a type of test called a perfusion study, which shows where the blood flow goes during these interventions.

Echocardiograms: This is a sonogram or ultrasound of your heart. It looks at the heart valves and the general ability of the heart to contract and pump blood. It's often used in conjunction with a treadmill test and/or medications to see how the heart pumps at higher rates.

CT Scan: A special type of CT scan examines the amount of calcium in the arteries supplying the heart. This helps determine whether plaque is present, since normal blood vessels do not contain calcium deposits. This is useful for at-risk women with heart disease symptoms. Research is ongoing to see how useful it is for detecting heart disease in women without any symptoms.

Guard Your Heart

I have to say it one more time: Heart disease is the number-one killer of women in the United States, so you need to consider yourself personally at risk and do everything in your power to reduce it. Creating healthy heart habits when you're in your thirties and forties can make a huge difference in your future health. Start now: The clock and your heart are ticking.

11

Boning Up

Preventing Osteoporosis

My patient Elyse is the picture of youth, vitality, and health at age forty-nine. She eats right, loves to exercise, and has a normal body weight. She looks and feels great, and so does her mother, Sharon, age eighty-nine.

When Elyse went through menopause this year, I sent her for a baseline bone density, or DEXA, scan, which I recommend for all my patients who have gone through menopause. Elyse's mom, who is also my patient, has osteoporosis, so I wanted to keep an eye on Elyse's bones over the coming years. Although national guidelines suggest bone scans starting at age sixty-five, I'd rather catch this bone disease in its early stages than find an advanced case fifteen years later.

When Elyse's scan results came back, I was shocked: At forty-nine, she had full-blown osteoporosis of her hip and spine.

Most of us think of osteoporosis as an old ladies' disease, something we shouldn't worry about in our thirties and forties. But as Elyse's case shows, younger women can and do get osteoporosis. Even if you're not one of these rare cases, if you start treating your bones well now, you can help stave off the disease and keep your body healthy, strong, and beautiful for decades to come.

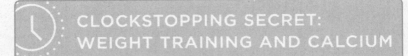

CLOCKSTOPPING SECRET: WEIGHT TRAINING AND CALCIUM

Osteoporosis is *not* an inevitable part of aging. About 55 percent of people over age fifty suffer from this debilitating condition, but there's a lot you can do to strengthen your bones and stave off the disease. Most important, you need to do weight-bearing exercise (running, weight lifting, yoga) several times a week starting in your thirties and forties. Start now: These measures won't work unless you begin them while you're still young.

No Bones About It:
The Dangers of Osteoporosis

Osteoporosis is a serious disease. It can cause painful fractures, often in the hips, wrists, or spine. It can disable you. It can even shorten your life.[1] One study found that older people with osteoporosis who broke a bone had a higher chance of dying in the next five to ten years than those who did not. People who had two fractures had a higher death rate within just five years. The good news is, there are things you can do now to lower your risk. But beware: These steps will help now, while you're young, but won't work as well later on.

To understand this disease, it helps to first appreciate the mysteries of the bone. You probably think of your bones as solid and unchanging, like the chassis of a car or the steel frame of a building. But that's not true: Bones are living, evolving tissue, constantly being broken down and built up in a process called remodeling. In fact, you can think of your bones as a house that's being continually rebuilt by two competing teams of workers. One team, the bone builder cells called osteoblasts, builds new bone. This team lays down new bone matrix, a network made up of collagen, salts, and other substances that form the foundation of bone.

The other team, the bone destroyer cells called osteoclasts, is the demolition crew. Osteoclasts destroy old bone to make room for new bone. At some stages in life, the builders pull ahead, and at others, the destroyers win. Whichever team is winning determines your bone density, or how strong your bones are. Osteoporosis happens when the demolition crew permanently overtakes the builders, and the result is weakened, porous bone, with low density and low mass. This weak and fragile bone is at risk for fractures, which can happen in any part of the skeleton, although the hips, spine, and wrists are the most common locations.

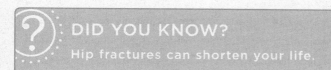

DID YOU KNOW?
Hip fractures can shorten your life.

Almost one in four people aged fifty and over will die in the year following a hip fracture.[2]

PAST YOUR PEAK

I hate to say this, since the overall message of this book is that you're really just reaching your peak in your thirties and forties (and, with a little luck, into your fifties and beyond if you follow the advice in this book!). But frankly, your bones really *are* past their prime, at least in terms of density. Women reach their maximum bone density between the ages of eighteen and twenty-five. That's the greatest bone mass you'll ever have—and I bet you never even knew you had it!

The good news is that if you exercised and got lots of calcium and vitamin D in your teens and early twenties, you laid down a lifetime foundation of dense bone.

After you reach twenty-five to thirty, you don't get to build up your density. You just preserve what you already have. Most of the time, your body does a pretty good job of that in your thirties and forties, thanks to the primary female hormone, estrogen. Both types of bone cells, osteoblasts and osteoclasts, have estrogen receptors. Estrogen turns on the bone builder cells, increasing their numbers and also increasing collagen production, important for laying down new bone matrix. Estrogen has the opposite effect on osteoclasts, the wrecking crew: It turns off the activity of bone reabsorption and shortens the life of these cells. The result is that you preserve your existing bone density despite the ongoing remodeling project.

In your teens and early twenties, you were making more bone than you destroyed. After menopause, or approximately around age fifty, you begin to lose more than you make. Your estrogen levels drop and no longer keep the wrecking crew in check. Seven years after menopause, you may have up to 20 percent less bone density than earlier in your life.[3] Fortunately, if you started out with more bone, you'll be less affected by this loss of strength. Your goal is to slow or prevent this process by keeping your bones as dense as possible for as long as possible. The time for that is now, while you're young, healthy, active, and have estrogen circulating in your body. There's no time to lose.

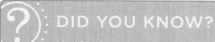

DID YOU KNOW?

Half of women will break bones after fifty.

Approximately one in two women over the age of fifty will have an osteoporosis-related fracture in their lifetime.[4]

The Body Beautiful Prescription: Protect Your Bones

Fortunately for your skeleton, there are several things that you can do to keep your bones strong and healthy and decrease your risk of bone loss.

1. STRESS YOUR MUSCLES

You've heard me sing the virtues of exercise in every single chapter so far, so I'm sure you're not surprised to hear that exercise helps your bones. But not just any kind of exercise will help your bones; you need a certain kind of activity that stresses them. Yep, in this case, stress is good, and I don't mean the kind of stress induced by your boss or your kids. I mean stress as in asking your bones to tolerate more force and mass. When you run, lift weights, or do other exercise that puts weight on your bones, the bones get stronger and lay down more bone matrix. Specifically, walking, jogging, aerobics, yoga, hiking, and lifting weights all force your muscles and tendons to pull on your bones. This pull is the force that stimulates the bone building cells to work harder. When osteoblasts work harder, your bones get stronger and you're less likely to suffer fractures as you age.

Note that I didn't put swimming on this list. It's a great way to condition your heart and burn calories, but it is *not* a weight-bearing exercise. By all means, swim to protect your heart, but remember to lift weights and jog to protect your bones.

DON'T WAIT FOR WEIGHTS!

As I said in chapter 2, lifting weights is one of the best exercises a woman can do. It won't bulk up your muscles, but it will help you burn more calories at rest and appear leaner. And it's absolutely great for your skeletal health! Lift weights two to three times a week for the optimum benefits.

2. EAT FOODS WITH CALCIUM AND VITAMIN D

To slow your loss of bone, you need to eat a diet full of calcium and vitamin D. If your body isn't getting enough calcium, it breaks down bones to get it, accelerating bone loss. Many of my patients tell me, "I get plenty of calcium! I drink lots of milk." But the truth is, they'd have to drink three or four glasses of milk a day to get the 1,000 mg of calcium recommended for women ages nineteen to fifty. More than 75 percent of Americans are calcium deficient, and most women underestimate their calcium needs by at least 50 percent.[5]

These are some of my favorite sources of calcium and vitamin D. Be sure that your diet includes some of these every day:

- Milk, cheese, yogurt, ice cream
- Green leafy vegetables such as spinach or kale
- Sardines
- Soybeans
- Fortified orange juice
- Fortified cereals

3. SUPPLEMENTS

With both calcium and vitamin D, it's best to get what you need from foods like those listed above. But supplements *in the right dose* can't hurt, and can help if you're not getting enough. In chapter 1, I recommend calcium and vitamin D supplements as part of the Five-Day/Two-Day Plan. Here's a quick reminder.

- **Calcium:** For healthy women ages thirty to fifty, I recommend 500 mg taken twice a day for a total of 1,000 mg a day (the body can't absorb more than 500–600 mg of calcium at a time). If you take thyroid medication, don't take it with calcium, which interferes with the absorption of the thyroid medicine. Wait two or three hours between taking them.
- **Vitamin D_3:** 1,000 IU per day. Because vitamin D_3 is fat soluble, it's best to take it with a meal.

Bones at Risk

Committing to weight-bearing exercise and making sure you get plenty of calcium and vitamin D can help keep your bones young. But you also need to understand the factors that might increase your risk of osteoporosis, and what kind of screening and medication can help. As with all diseases, some factors are under your control, and some aren't. It's important to know the difference and control what you can.

RISK FACTORS BEYOND YOUR CONTROL

Age
Osteoporosis is common among older people, although not everyone gets it. And as with Elyse, you don't have to be old to already have weak bones.

Gender
Women are more likely to get osteoporosis than men, perhaps because women have smaller, weaker, thinner bones to begin with. But men can get it, too. An estimated one out of four men over fifty will break a bone due to osteoporosis. A man fifty years old or older is more likely to have an osteoporosis fracture than he is to get prostate cancer.[6]

Menopause
The earlier you go through menopause, the greater your risk for osteoporosis, since the level of estrogen circulating in your blood drops.

Family History
Like so many medical and health issues, your family history plays a significant role in determining your risk for osteoporosis. If your mother or father had osteoporosis, a curving or hunched spine, or broken bones later in life, you are at increased risk yourself.

ARE YOUR BONES SICK, TOO?

Certain chronic illnesses or conditions can also increase your risk of osteoporosis. If you have any of these conditions, talk to your doctor about whether your bones might be at risk. These include:

- cancer
- chronic lung disease
- liver or kidney disease
- irritable bowel syndrome
- rheumatoid arthritis
- low thyroid (hypothyroidism)

RISKS YOU CONTROL

The great news: You can do a lot to reduce your risk of osteoporosis now, while you're young. We've already discussed the importance of weight-bearing exercise and diet, but there are a few other lifestyle issues that you can affect.

Smoking

Smoking is bad for your bones (and your lungs, heart, skin, teeth, brain, etc.). Smoking generates substances known as free radicals, which kill osteoblasts (the bone builders), harm the blood vessels that supply nourishment to your bones, and damage cells throughout the body. These damaged cells create a domino effect, increasing the stress hormone cortisol, which leads to bone destruction. Smoking in your forties and fifties accelerates the bone loss that occurs during the normal aging process. So there's yet another reason to quit smoking immediately.

Alcohol

Although we don't fully understand why, too much alcohol is toxic to bone-building cells. Drinking more than a moderate amount (more than a drink a day, or seven a week) may also affect hormone production by altering liver function, hormonal balance, and calcium and vitamin D metabolism.[7]

However, here's an interesting exception: In women who have already gone through menopause, moderate alcohol intake may be associated with an *increase* in bone density, though more research is needed. Given other research into the potentially beneficial impact of red wine on the heart, some patients take research as a license to start drinking, or to drink more. The truth is, if you don't drink, you shouldn't start just because of the research. If you do, keep your alcohol consumption to moderate levels.

Your Body Shape

Although being too thin can be a risk factor for weak bones, new research suggests that fat carried around the waistline may also put your bones at risk. A preliminary study of young women who had not yet gone through menopause found that those with a body shaped like an apple had lower bone density.[8]

Low Estrogen Levels

Some women with irregular periods suffer from low estrogen levels, which can weaken bones. This often happens in women who are very thin, have lost a great deal of weight, or who do strenuous exercise. It is also common in women with eating disorders such as anorexia nervosa. Some athletes experience what doctors call the athletic triad: low body weight, no periods, low bone mass. If you have irregular periods due to low estrogen levels, talk to your doctor about how this may affect your bones and what you can do about it. Sometimes a low-dose birth control pill can provide part of the supplementary estrogen that your bones need.

Medications

Some medications, including antiseizure drugs, blood thinners, steroids, and some breast cancer drugs, increase your risk of osteoporosis. This isn't exactly a lifestyle choice: With medication like this, if you need it, you need it. But you should talk to your doctor about the impact your medications may have on your bones, and take steps to reduce your risk through exercise and other measures listed here.

DRUGS AFFECTING BONE DENSITY
- Anticonvulsants
- Steroids (when taken for more than three months)
- Blood thinners like heparin or Lovenox
- Thyroid medication
- Lithium
- Proton pump inhibitors (to block stomach acid)
- Certain antibiotics (such as tetracycline)
- Methotrexate
- Depo-Provera (injectable contraception)
- Aromatase inhibitors, including Arimidex, Femara, and Aromasin, prescribed for breast cancer

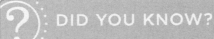

DID YOU KNOW?

Osteoporosis affects younger women (and men), too.

Although osteoporosis is most common in the elderly, it can also affect women in their thirties and forties, and even teenagers. It also affects men: About 20 percent of patients with osteoporosis are male.[9]

How Dense Are You? (Your Bones, I Mean)

It's easy to screen for bone density. A specialized X-ray called a DEXA measures your bone density at various sites in your body, usually your wrist, hip, and lumbar spine. You get three scores: overall bone mineral density (BMD), a Z-score (which compares your bone density to what's normal for people your age), and a T-score (used to diagnose osteoporosis in postmenopausal women over fifty).

Typically, women with risk factors have bone density screenings after menopause, and DEXAs are recommended for all women over the age of sixty-five. But I recommend my patients have a baseline DEXA at age fifty. If the results are normal, the test doesn't need to be repeated for another two years. If it shows osteoporosis, you may need to take a medication, and your tests should be repeated regularly to monitor the progress of the disease.

Midway between normal and full-blown osteoporosis lies osteopenia, a precursor to osteoporosis. Approximately 18 million people in the United States have osteopenia. If not caught early and treated aggressively with weight-bearing exercise and calcium and vitamin D_3 supplements, it can evolve into serious bone disease. If your DEXA scan shows osteopenia, your doctor will talk to you about treatment, and repeat the scan every one to two years.

Usually we don't screen women younger than fifty for osteoporosis (even though this helped my patient Elyse). The problem is, the medications used to treat osteoporosis are not recommended or approved for use by women of reproductive age, because they stay in the body for ten years or more and their safety during pregnancy has not been established. In addition, DEXA scans can underestimate bone density in young women who are slim and have a small body size, giving a false positive for osteopenia. So the general thinking is, why do the test if you can't treat the results?

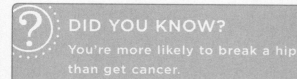

DID YOU KNOW?

You're more likely to break a hip than get cancer.

A woman's risk of an osteoporosis-related hip fracture is equal to her risk for breast, uterine, and ovarian cancers combined.[10]

Osteoporosis Medication

Osteoporosis medications are only approved for women who have gone through menopause, since they stay in your body for so long and may affect future pregnancies in ways we don't understand. Most women reading this book won't be able to take it, but if you went through menopause before fifty-one and bone scans show you have weak bones, it may be an option for you. The main class of drugs that slow or prevent osteoporosis is called bisphosphonates. Sold under the brand names of

Fosamax, Actonel, and Boniva, these drugs work by slowing the behavior of the bone-destroying osteoclast cells.

These drugs have several potential problems. One is that most of these medications can irritate your stomach and esophagus. To avoid that, you have to remain in an upright position for thirty minutes after taking the pill and before eating or drinking anything. Plus, some women taking these medications can experience a rare type of fracture in the thigh bone where dull, achy pain begins in the groin or thigh weeks or months before the femur actually breaks. The FDA recommends that people taking bisphosphonates for more than five years reevaluate the need for continued treatment with their doctor.[11]

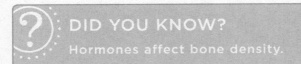

DID YOU KNOW?
Hormones affect bone density.

Your parathyroid hormone (not thyroid, but *para*thyroid) can affect your bone health. If you have weak bones, ask your doctor whether testing your PTH level may be necessary. Some doctors specialize in bone diseases and these hormonal conditions, so if you have unexplained osteoporosis, find a specialist in this area.

Build, Don't Break

The last word on bone health is, start now. If you wait until menopause, it's too late to minimize bone damage. Start lifting those weights, taking those supplements, and aggressively working to build your bones now, before it's too late. Bone up now, so your bones don't let you down later.

12

On the Attack: Arming Yourself Against Cancer

n the past thirty years, there's been a revolution in cancer treatment. Many types of cancer are no longer viewed as a death sentence. Instead, we think of these cancers like any other disease: conditions you can fight, survive, and, very often, live with for a long time. For some types of breast, uterine, thyroid, and skin cancers, the odds of survival are better than they've ever been.

This is all good news. But it also means more responsibility for you, as you develop the lifetime habits that will keep your body beautiful, strong, and healthy. Women today need to be more vigilant than ever about understanding how to lower their cancer risks and detect symptoms early. In chapter 9, we discussed breast cancer. Here are other important cancers for women to guard against.

How Cancer Works

To reduce your risk of all types of cancer, you first need to understand a little about the normal life cycle of a cell. Most cells in our body go through a circular life cycle that includes a resting stage, a growth phase, a replication stage, a checkpoint phase before cell division, and then a cell division stage. Also, most cells have a death phase; many cells are programmed to die to make room for new cells or at the end of their life cycles.

Cancer is the uncontrolled growth of abnormal, or malignant, cells. It develops when something in a cell's replication cycle has gone awry; a malignant cell is born and cell division occurs without any regulation. One malignant cell becomes two, two become four, and so on and so on, forming tumors. Through a process called metastasis, these cells sometimes move from one organ to another, or to other parts of the body, and can spread through the bloodstream and to lymph nodes.

CLOCKSTOPPING SECRET: MANY CANCERS ARE PREVENTABLE

You can stop the clock on many cancers simply by living a healthy life. A whopping 30–50 percent of cancer deaths are linked to lifestyle and behavior choices, like smoking, obesity, lack of exercise, having unprotected sex, and so on.[1]

Many factors can trigger cancer. Some of these factors are under our control, some are not. Your mission is to understand your risks for the most common cancers today and how to reduce those risks. In the rest of this chapter, I'll describe the most common types of cancer for women, including their symptoms, risk factors, screening methods, and protective steps you can take. But first, I want you to understand seven common symptoms that you should never ignore, symptoms that could help identify cancers early, but often go unreported. I don't want you to be alarmed, but I *do* want you to talk to your doctor if you're experiencing any of these. Better safe than sorry!

THE MOST COMMONLY IGNORED SYMPTOMS OF CANCER

Pain

Women are a stoic bunch. We handle monthly cramps, pregnancy, childbirth, maybe a kidney stone or two. (I've had these—and they were much more painful than childbirth!) So pain is something we often don't pay a lot of attention to, figuring it will go away. But persistent pain, even if it's vague in nature, can be an early symptom of certain types of cancer. These include uterine, ovarian, esophageal, pancreatic, and colorectal cancers. If you have any pain for more than two weeks, see your doctor. Your doctor will ask what makes the pain better or worse, how often it comes, the character or quality of the pain (constant, intermittent, dull, sharp), whether it radiates or travels to another location in your body, and how bad it is (usually on a scale of one to ten, with ten being the worst).

Blood in Your Stool, Urine, or Phlegm

You should not have blood in any of these bodily fluids. It may not be cancer—it could be an infection—but you should talk to your doctor. It's always a good idea to check both what's on the toilet paper and what's in the toilet bowl after you have a bowel movement or urinate. If you don't have your period and you see blood on the toilet paper, whether it comes from the vagina, bladder, or rectum, tell your doctor. Similarly, if you cough up blood, you need to talk to your doctor. It could be anything from an infection to lung cancer.

Change in Bowel or Bladder Habits

Sometimes an increase in urination is caused by a bladder or urinary tract infection, but it can also be a symptom of ovarian cancer. A change in your stool can indicate colon cancer. If you notice your trips to the bathroom are increasing, let your doctor know.

Unexplained Weight Loss

It's no wonder this symptom too often goes unreported. So many people are trying to lose weight that they don't always notice effortless weight loss. And if they *do* notice, they don't think it's a bad thing. But the truth is, losing weight without decreasing your calories or increasing your exercise could be a sign of cancer. If you notice your clothes getting looser or you lose more than eight to ten pounds in one month without trying, see your doctor.

Irregular Vaginal Bleeding

I always tell my patients that their periods and their regularity should be like a vital sign, just like blood pressure or heart rate. If your period is always regular, and suddenly you notice spotting in between periods or particularly heavy periods, this could indicate a cancer of the uterus. If this happens for a few months in a row, talk to your gynecologist. While hormonal conditions and even infections can cause irregular bleeding, it's important to exclude cancer as soon as you can.

Bloating

Many women feel bloated every month before or during their period—but that feeling should last only a few days. Bloating that occurs every day or that lasts for more than two weeks can signal ovarian cancer, especially if it happens along with pelvic pain and increased urination. Do not ignore increased feelings of bloating. Talk to your doctor, who may want you to see both a gynecologist and a gastroenterologist (GI specialist) during the course of the workup.

Indigestion

If you experience persistent indigestion discomfort in your chest, upper abdomen, or back, see your doctor. While heartburn can be triggered by food, excess weight, or some medications like Advil or Motrin, the same sensation can be a sign of cancer of the stomach or esophagus. Pain occurring in your upper back that comes after eating may be related to your pancreas. Talk to your doctor about ongoing indigestion symptoms.

Cough

Obviously, colds and allergies can cause a cough; so can some medications or GERD (heartburn). But a chronic cough lasting more than two weeks can be a symptom of lung cancer, especially if you smoke, used to smoke, or live with a smoker. Report this to your doctor.

Other Red Flags

Fever, vague abdominal pain, skin or breast changes, fatigue, trouble swallowing, or visible changes inside your mouth can all be signs or symptoms of cancer. Again, I don't want to alarm you. Most of the time, these simply signal other, noncancerous conditions. In medicine, we often say, "When you hear hooves outside the door, think of horses, not zebras." In other words, common symptoms usually mean common maladies. Don't assume the worst, but don't ignore these warning signs, either. Talk to your doctor: You have nothing to lose and lots to gain—like maybe saving your life.[2]

The Seven Most Common Cancers for Women

In addition to the common symptoms above, each type of cancer has its own unique signs, as well as its own risk factors and preventive measures. To keep your body beautiful and strong, you need to understand the symptoms, your personal risks, and what you can do to reduce them.

LUNG CANCER

My husband, Rob, is a surgeon who specializes in treating lung cancer, so this topic is very important to my family. It should be important to you, too, because no cancer kills more women than lung cancer. In fact, it kills more women than breast, uterine, and ovarian cancers *combined*. Every year, seventy-one thousand women in the United States die from lung cancer. That's more than a quarter of all cancer deaths among women.

Here's another striking fact about lung cancer: One in five women with lung cancer *have never smoked*. This means that while 80 percent of women with lung cancer were or are smokers, 20 percent have lung cancer that was not caused by smoking. So even if you've never smoked, you can't assume you won't get it.

> ## ? DID YOU KNOW?
> Lung cancer kills more women than any other cancer.
>
> One in sixteen women will develop lung cancer in her lifetime, and roughly 9 percent of women diagnosed with lung cancer are younger than fifty years of age.[3] More women die from lung cancer than from breast, uterine, and ovarian cancers put together.

Risk Factors

Smoking. This is the number-one risk factor for lung cancer. Every single cigarette you smoke contains thousands of carcinogens—chemicals known to cause cancer. And every single cigarette you smoke damages cells in your body, in both your lungs and your blood vessels.

Secondhand and thirdhand smoke. You don't have to smoke to be hurt by carcinogens in cigarettes. Considerable evidence shows that exposure to smoke (for example, living, working, or sitting in a car with someone who smokes) is also dangerous. One study showed that people who are exposed to secondhand smoke increase their risk of developing lung cancer by almost 30 percent.[4] Thirdhand smoke—that smoky smell that lingers in the clothes and hair of smokers, as well as upholstery, carpets, and other items—also contains carcinogens and presents a significant health risk.[5]

Environmental toxins. Exposure to environmental toxins including radon, asbestos, air pollution, and certain types of industrial chemicals can also increase your risk of lung cancer.

Family history. Some people are genetically predisposed to getting lung cancer, so be sure to tell your doctor if anyone in your family has had lung cancer.

Hormones. Some research indicates that there may be a hormonal factor at play for women with lung cancer, and that women who take hormone replacement therapy after menopause may be at increased risk.

Symptoms

- Persistent cough
- Shortness of breath
- Hoarseness
- Change in phlegm or sputum production or color
- Chest or back pain
- Weight loss

Screening

Catching lung cancer early can save lives. When lung cancer is diagnosed at an early stage, half of patients are still alive five years later. When diagnosed at a later stage, though, lung cancer kills 98 percent of patients within that time frame. So if you're at risk, careful screening is critical.

Until recently, doctors relied on simple chest X-rays to screen for lung cancer, looking for tiny spots on the lungs. But in 2010, a landmark study revealed that using CT scans (computerized tomography scans, which take a series of imaged "slices" of our body to produce cross-sectional pictures) could save lives by helping doctors detect cancer as small as 2–3 millimeters in size (while chest X-rays usually only spot tumors that are an inch or more in size). If your doctor recommends an X-ray, ask about having a CT scan instead.

If you have any symptoms of lung cancer, your doctor may also recommend other screening tests, including an analysis of your sputum.

Prevention

You can decrease the risk of lung cancer by:

- Never smoking cigarettes, cigars, or pipes
- Quitting smoking
- Avoiding secondhand smoke
- Limiting alcohol
- Exercising
- Eating more fruits and vegetables[6]

A BREATHALYZER FOR LUNG CANCER?

Exciting new research is now under way to see if cancer can be detected simply by analyzing your exhaled breath.[7] Cancer cells make different volatile organic compounds (by-products of metabolism produced by cells) than healthy cells, and researchers are developing new tests to identify these biomarkers and lung cancer.

QUIT NOW: IT'S NOT TOO LATE

If you quit smoking and are smoke-free for more than ten years, you can cut your odds of developing lung cancer by 50 percent, according to the American Cancer Society.

COLORECTAL CANCER

Colorectal cancer, which includes colon cancer and rectal cancer, is the number-three cancer killer among women, behind lung and breast cancer. An estimated 101,700 new cases of colon cancer and almost forty thousand new cases of rectal cancer are diagnosed in the United States each year. You have about a one in twenty chance of developing colorectal cancer in your lifetime (men have a slightly higher risk). Fortunately, campaigns by celebrities like Katie Couric have raised public awareness about this common killer, and the death rate from colorectal cancer is declining, probably due to earlier detection and better treatment.[8]

Risk Factors

   Family history. As many as 20 percent of people who are diagnosed
      with colorectal cancer have a relative with the same disease. If the
      person in your family with colorectal cancer is a first-degree rela-
      tive (your parent, child, or sibling), your risk of developing cancer
      of the colon is roughly doubled. If you know that you have a rela-
      tive with colorectal cancer, try to collect as much information as
      possible about his or her disease. Your doctor will want to know
      how old he or she was when diagnosed, what stage the cancer was
      at, and what the treatment was.
   Age. The chances of getting colorectal cancer increase as we age.
      More than 90 percent of those diagnosed are over fifty. (Of course,
      that means that 10 percent of patients are under fifty, so don't
      dismiss risk factors or symptoms just because you're still young.)
   Race and ethnicity. African-Americans have higher rates of colon
      cancer than other racial groups, and Jews with eastern European
      ancestry have higher rates than other ethnic groups.
   Irritable bowel disease or other bowel issues. A history of

bowel trouble, including colorectal polyps, Crohn's disease, ulcerative colitis, or irritable bowel disease (this is different from IBS, or irritable bowel syndrome), places you at increased risk of cancer. Researchers believe that chronic inflammation of the colon due to these conditions can cause the cells that line the colon to evolve into malignant cells. Good news, though: There is no evidence that IBS increases the risk of colorectal cancer.

Genetic syndromes. Affecting approximately 5–10 percent of people with cancer of the colon or rectum, a number of genetic syndromes are associated with increased risk of colorectal cancer, including:

FAP: familial adenomatous polyposis
HNPCC: hereditary nonpolyposis colon cancer
Peutz-Jeghers syndrome
MUTYH-associated polyposis
Turcot syndrome

DID YOU KNOW?
Most intestinal polyps are not cancer.

Cancer is present in only about 5 percent of intestinal polyps.[9]

DID YOU KNOW?
Smokers are more likely to die from colorectal cancer than nonsmokers.

Women who smoke are 40 percent more likely to die of colorectal cancer than nonsmokers. Yet another reason to kick butt![10]

Symptoms
- Blood in your stool (don't assume it's from hemorrhoids)
- Abdominal pain
- Unexplained weight loss
- Change in the caliber or appearance of your stool
- Change in frequency of bowel movements
- Rectal pain or pressure
- Bloating
- Iron-deficiency anemia
- Fatigue

Screening
The really amazing thing about screening for colorectal cancer is that the same process that can identify potential problems can also treat them. If a colonoscopy detects a small growth called a precancerous polyp, it can be removed then and there. That's great news, because colorectal cancer is one form of cancer that follows a well-understood (and often slow) progression, from the growth of a precancerous polyp to a malignant lesion. If the polyp is caught early, cancer can actually be prevented.

Even if cancer is already present, though, finding and treating it early, before it spreads through the lining of the colon, makes a big difference in survival rates. That's why colorectal cancer screening is so important. If you're at average risk, the American Cancer Society recommends that screening start at age fifty with a colonoscopy. If the results are normal, the test doesn't need to be repeated for another ten years. If you have any risk factors for colorectal cancer, screening starts earlier, at forty or younger, and is repeated more frequently. There are many other screening methods besides colonoscopy, including flexible sigmoidoscopy, double-contrast barium enemas, fecal occult blood testing, fecal immunochemical testing, and stool DNA testing. Your doctor can take you through the pros and cons of each to help you make the best choice.

Prevention

You can reduce your risk for colorectal cancer in several ways. And guess what? They prevent lots of other diseases as well. Many of these will also lower your chances of developing type 2 diabetes, which has been associated with a higher risk of colorectal cancer.

- Eat a diet low in red, processed, or charbroiled meats and high in fruits, vegetables, and fiber.
- Exercise.
- Maintain a healthy, non-obese body weight.
- Quit smoking.
- Limit your alcohol consumption.
- Consider taking aspirin daily.

Recent studies have shown that for some people, taking a low dose of aspirin reduced the risk of developing colon cancer by 24 percent. However, because aspirin can cause some potentially serious side effects, like internal bleeding, the American Cancer Society is not yet recommending that people take it purely to reduce colon cancer risk.[11]

THYROID CANCER

When I discuss thyroid cancer in women with my surgeon friend Dr. Steven Libutti, director of the Montefiore Einstein Center for Cancer Care, he gets very excited. He feels that thyroid cancer in women is an opportunity for a real cancer triumph. This one can be found, treated, and cured. When diagnosed early, more than 97 percent of patients with thyroid cancer are still alive five years later.

But Steven and I still worry. The problem isn't the cancer itself. It's that so many women and their doctors are not on the lookout for it. We *should* be. More than thirty-four thousand women in the United States are diagnosed with thyroid cancer each year, and nearly 66 percent of cases are detected in women between the ages of twenty and fifty-five. The incidence of thyroid cancer in the United States is increasing, though we don't fully understand why. The rate has nearly doubled since 1990.[12]

Risk Factors

Gender. Women are two to three times more likely than men to get this disease.

Age. Though the risk of many cancers increases with age, thyroid cancer is often referred to as a young person's cancer, with most cases being diagnosed before a person's seventh decade.

Ethnicity. Caucasian and Asian women are more likely than other races to develop thyroid cancer, though a person of any race can be affected.

Family history. A family history of thyroid cancer, polyps, or goiters increases the risk of cancer. Also, some hereditary conditions increase the risk of thyroid cancer, including some tied to gynecologic conditions. These include women with Carney complex type 1 (which involves many dark skin lesions all over the body, heart problems, breast fibroadenomas, and hormonal issues) and those with Cowden's disease (which is associated with an increased risk of uterine, breast, and thyroid cancers).

Environmental factors. Radiation exposure or a diet that is low in iodine can increase the risk of thyroid cancer. In the United States, these factors are less common today than they were in the past.

Symptoms
- A lump in the neck or throat
- Pain in the neck or throat
- Hoarseness or a change in your voice
- A persistent cough
- Difficulty swallowing or breathing

Screening
There is no general screening test for thyroid cancer, but there are ways to detect it. Typically, a patient or her doctor actually feels a lump in the patient's throat. Next, an imaging test, such as an ultrasound, CT scan, or MRI is ordered to determine if there's a potentially cancerous mass present. If so, it is biopsied, sometimes with surgery, but often with a syringe, called a fine needle aspiration (FNA). Blood tests are often part of this workup to help distinguish between a goiter (thyroid dysfunction) and a malignancy.

Prevention
The best you can do to reduce your risk of thyroid cancer is to avoid radiation exposure and to be aware of your own body so you can alert your doctor if you feel a lump or bump in your throat.

SKIN CANCER/MELANOMA
Skin cancer is the sixth most common cancer in the United States, with more than one million cases diagnosed every year. While there are several forms of skin cancer, the most deadly form is known as malignant melanoma. It arises in the pigment-producing cells of the skin, known as melanocytes. This cancer can strike at any age. More than one-third

of malignant melanoma cases occur in people under fifty-five, and the incidence among young women is on the rise.

Because melanoma is more deadly than the other types of skin cancer (such as basal cell carcinoma and squamous cell carcinoma), prevention, screening, and early detection are key for survival.

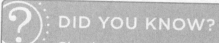

DID YOU KNOW?

Check your upper back and legs for cancer.

The most common sites for malignant melanoma in women are the upper back and legs.[13]

Risk Factors

I'm at risk for melanoma. I have freckles, many moles, blond hair, and spent my teenage summers in the sun, working as a lifeguard. So I'm vigilant about having skin checks at least once a year. You should be, too, especially if you share any of these risk factors.

- **Your coloring.** People with fair skin, blond or red hair, and blue eyes are at increased risk, as is anyone who burns easily and is sensitive to the sun.
- **Race.** Caucasians are twenty times more likely than African-Americans to develop melanoma.[14] But even if you have dark skin, you can still get it.
- **Moles.** People with fifty or more moles on their bodies are at higher risk.
- **Sunburns.** People with a history of bad sunburns or the use of tanning beds are at increased risk of melanoma.
- **Family history.** If you have relatives who have had melanoma, or you have had other types of skin cancer or have a weakened im-

mune system (especially from breast or thyroid cancer), your risk
for melanoma is increased.

Xeroderma pigmentosum. In this genetic condition, cells are
unable to repair damage from ultraviolet rays and cancer risk is
increased.

SYMPTOMS: THE ABCDEs OF MELANOMA

The acronym ABCDE is helpful in remembering the signs of skin
cancer.

A **is for** *asymmetry*. A mole should look the same on both sides if you
were to draw an imaginary line through its center. An asymmetrical
mole may be cancerous.

B **is for** *border*. The border of a mole should be smooth and regular, not
jagged.

C **is for** *color*. The color of the mole should be the same throughout.

D **is for** *diameter*. A mole should not be larger than the size of a pencil
eraser.

E **is for** *evolving*. Any mole that is changing in any way should be evaluated by a dermatologist.

In addition, you might feel itching, bleeding, or pain.

Screening

- Skin check: As part of a routine exam, your doctor should inspect
  your skin, head to foot, looking for suspicious moles like I've described above.
- Self-check: You should do your own skin checks regularly, scan-
  ning every inch of your skin for signs.

? DID YOU KNOW?

Skin cancer can still occur where the sun doesn't shine.

Skin cancer can develop anywhere, even though sun-exposed areas on the body are the most common. Don't forget hard-to-see spots like the scalp, fingernails, in between your fingers and toes, and your genital region. If you can't see these areas yourself, ask your partner to check them regularly, and see a doctor for official regular examinations.

Prevention

The best way to reduce your risk of melanoma is to be diligent about protecting your skin from the harmful UV rays of the sun. Although you may hear some health experts talk about how the sun is a good source of natural vitamin D, remember you can get plenty of vitamin D in food and supplements instead of sun exposure. As the American Academy of Dermatology says, "A tan is not a sign of good health. It's a sign that you've damaged your skin." To protect your skin:

- Use sunscreen daily. Choose a sunscreen of at least SPF 30 that blocks both UVA and UVB rays.
- Apply sunscreen all over your body, not just on the areas that will be directly exposed to the sun's rays, at least twenty minutes before going outside. Use as much sunscreen as would fit in a shot glass.
- Reapply every two hours when you're in the sun.
- Wear a hat and sunglasses that wrap around and protect the sides of your eyes.
- Limit your time outside during the hours from 10 a.m. to 4 p.m., when the sun is strongest.

? DID YOU KNOW?
Tanning beds increase cancer risk.

The use of indoor tanning beds increases your risk of melanoma by 75 percent.[15]

OVARIAN CANCER

The deadliest of all gynecological cancers, ovarian cancer kills about fifteen thousand women a year. Part of the problem is that tumors can grow quite large and spread widely in the pelvic and abdominal cavities before they are detected. More than 50 percent of women with ovarian cancer are not diagnosed until the disease has reached advanced stages. So even though the chance of developing ovarian cancer (about one in seventy-one) is relatively small compared to other cancers, it's important to understand your risk factors and how to avoid this disease.[16]

Risk Factors

Age. Most ovarian cancer develops in women over the age of forty-five, with the average age at diagnosis approximately sixty. Younger women also get ovarian cancer. About 7 percent of cases are diagnosed in women aged thirty-five to forty-four.[17] Younger women with ovarian cancer face better odds than women who are over the age of sixty-five when their cancer is detected.

Family history. If you have a first-degree relative (mother, sister, or daughter) with the disease, your chances of developing ovarian cancer are about one in twenty.

Genetics. If you carry the BRCA mutation, which we discussed in chapter 9, your risk of developing ovarian cancer is increased. Roughly 11–15 percent of ovarian cancer cases are due to the BRCA mutation.[18] If one of your parents has the BRCA mutation, you have a 50 percent chance of having it as well. Also, if your family has a history of breast cancer at a young age or if you're of eastern European Jewish ancestry, you are at increased risk of the BRCA mutation. Talk to your doctor about getting tested for the mutation. In addition, women with hereditary nonpolyposis colorectal cancer (HNPCC) are at increased risk of ovarian cancer.

Breast cancer. Talk about unfair. If you've had breast cancer before the age of forty, your risk of ovarian cancer is higher.

No pregnancies or other uninterrupted ovulation. If you've never been pregnant, never been on birth control pills, had your first period before age twelve, or went through menopause after age fifty, your ovarian cancer risk is higher because of uninterrupted ovulation. One theory is that one form of ovarian cancer is caused by constant, prolonged, or excessive damage to the outer surface of the ovaries, and since ovulation ruptures follicles in the ovaries, decades of these ruptures with no break may lead to cancer.

Symptoms

Ovarian cancer's symptoms are very common and somewhat vague, so you may feel silly asking your doctor about them. But if you have these symptoms for more than two weeks, see your gynecologist. Because many of these symptoms are associated with the digestive tract, he or she may also recommend a gastrointestinal workup *in addition to* performing a thorough gynecological exam and sonogram. I ask my patients at every visit about these symptoms, and your doctor should ask you, too.

- Bloating for more than two weeks
- Pelvic pain or pressure
- More frequent urination
- Early satiety (feeling full after eating very little)
- Increasing abdominal girth
- Weight loss or weight gain
- Indigestion
- General feeling that something isn't right

Screening

Unfortunately, there is no simple, accurate screening test for ovarian cancer. In addition, we can't do a biopsy on the ovaries without doing major surgery requiring general anesthesia. This means that, for now, we have to do the best we can to identify women at high risk of ovarian cancer, or who are having signs or symptoms that may indicate ovarian cancer. Currently, this is done based on a patient's medical history, pelvic exam, blood tests, and pelvic sonogram.

Pelvic exam: In adult women, a proper gynecologic exam involves *both* a vaginal examination and a rectovaginal exam. The doctor inserts the index finger into the vagina and the middle finger of the same hand into the rectum. This is the only way to examine the ovaries and pelvis thoroughly, since when you lie down on the exam table, your ovaries can flop backward and fall behind the uterus. As uncomfortable as this type of exam may be, remember that it's important for your health.

Blood tests: Blood tests can detect substances that serve as markers for ovarian tumors—clues that tumors may be present. One of those markers is CA-125, a protein that's elevated in approximately 85 percent of women with one type of ovarian cancer. Unfortunately, CA-125 can also be elevated when there's no cancer, or it can be normal when there *is* cancer, especially in early stages.[19] So, to say the least, this is not a perfect test. If your doctor recommends this one, be prepared for uncertain results. The test is more useful for women after menopause, because certain conditions like pregnancy that cause elevated CA-125 are no longer a concern. Other markers of ovarian cancer include HE4, AFP, LDH, HCG, and inhibin. The blood test for HE4 can be particularly helpful in premenopausal women with a mass on sonogram who are being screened for ovarian cancer.

Pelvic sonogram: If your doctor detects a mass during a pelvic exam, if you have a family history of ovarian cancer, or if you're having pelvic pain or bloating, your doctor may order a pelvic ultrasound. Not every mass on your ovary means cancer. It could well be a noncancerous cyst. Especially in women who are still getting a period, ovaries make cysts for a living—during ovulation, ovaries literally make cysts, which burst to release eggs. Sometimes normal cysts become quite large. If the sonogram shows a cyst, your doctor may repeat the ultrasound in four to eight weeks, or draw blood markers or obtain a CT scan or MRI for more information.

OVARIAN CANCER: FIND THE RIGHT SURGEON

Your chances for survival of ovarian cancer improve if you have your initial surgery with a gynecologic oncologist. Though many general gynecologists can perform an initial surgery to remove the ovaries and/or uterus, the best surgery for ovarian cancer is highly specialized and should be performed by a board-certified gyn-oncology surgeon. Al-

though some general ob-gyns will tell their patients they can do the surgery and have a second operation later if they need it, that's not the best
treatment and can lower survival rates. This is not a surgery you have to
rush, so you can take the time to find the right surgeon.

Prevention

As scary as ovarian cancer sounds, there's good news: There are several
effective strategies you can use to reduce your risk.

A healthy lifestyle. As with other cancers, a diet high in fruits and
vegetables and a healthy body weight help reduce your risk of
ovarian cancer.

Birth control pills. Women who have taken the pill for at least
three years reduce their risk of ovarian cancer by nearly 60 percent. What's more, this risk reduction continues even after women
stop taking the pill.[20] The pill works to prevent ovarian cancer by
suppressing the activity and ovulation process of the ovaries, reducing the chance of damage to the outer surface of the ovarian
capsule.

Tied tubes. Having your tubes tied (ligation of the fallopian tubes)
is another way to reduce your risk of developing ovarian cancer
after you're done having kids.

Ovary removal. Removal of both ovaries can reduce the risk of
ovarian cancer considerably, although it's still possible to develop
a cancer that resembles ovarian cancer (called PPC). Occasionally, if a woman has the BRCA mutation and therefore a high risk
of ovarian cancer, removing ovaries as a preventive measure can
save her life. However, women who have their ovaries removed
prophylactically, when there is no cancer present, are more likely

to have a shorter life expectancy due to death from cardiovascular causes. Therefore, you have to weigh the risks carefully.

UTERINE CANCER

Uterine cancer is the fourth most common cancer among women. In 2010, almost forty-three thousand women in the United States were diagnosed with uterine cancer. Almost eight thousand women die of the disease every year. The predominant type of uterine cancer is called endometrial cancer, since the cancer develops in the endometrium—the inner layer of the uterus.

Risk Factors

Age. Uterine cancer is most common in women who are over the age of fifty, and the average age at the time of diagnosis is sixty. Only thirty-six out of a hundred thousand women ages forty to forty-nine get uterine cancer.

Race. Caucasian women are more likely to get uterine cancer than African-American women, but African-American women are more likely to die of it. Possible reasons for this are that women of color tend to get more aggressive types of uterine cancer and/ or may get less prompt treatment.

Obesity. If you're obese, you're more prone to uterine cancer, as well as many other diseases.

Cancer treatment. Some cancer treatments increase your risk of uterine cancer, including the breast cancer drug tamoxifen and radiation therapy for pelvic cancer.

Hormone therapy. Women who have taken hormone therapy called unopposed estrogen are at increased risk. This kind of hormone treatment can trigger a process called endometrial hyper-plasia, which can progress to uterine cancer if left untreated.

Never having been pregnant. Pregnancy protects women against uterine cancer.

Irregular periods. If you have irregular periods (especially if you're obese), your risk of uterine cancer may be higher.

Symptoms

- Irregular vaginal bleeding, spotting, or discharge
- Pelvic pain
- Change in bladder patterns
- Deep pelvic pain during intercourse

Screening

There is no generally accepted screening test for uterine cancer. If you have symptoms, your doctor can do a simple endometrial biopsy in the office. Your doctor may also recommend a dilation and curettage, where part of the uterine lining is removed, or a hysteroscopy, where a small camera is passed through the cervix and looks directly into the uterus. In addition, imaging tests like sonograms, CT scans, or MRIs can also be helpful, depending on the individual case.

Prevention

The same factors that protect against ovarian cancer also protect against uterine cancer, including overall health, diet, weight, and taking the pill.[21]

CERVICAL CANCER

The cervix is the lower part of the uterus. I often tell my patients that it serves as the gatekeeper between the vagina and the uterus, choosing whether to allow sperm or bacteria in, and letting blood and babies out. Each year in the United States, there are over twelve thousand cases of cervical cancer diagnosed and approximately four thousand deaths due to the disease. Half of all women diagnosed with cervical cancer are younger than forty-seven years of age. In Africa, cervical cancer is the leading cause of cancer death among women. Almost all cases of cervical cancer worldwide are caused by HPV, the sexually transmitted human papillomavirus.

Risk Factors

In addition to smoking, a poor diet, and a family history of cervical cancer, risk factors include:

Sexual habits. Women who had sexual intercourse at a young age or have had a lot of sexual partners are at higher risk for cervical cancer.

HIV/AIDS. Having HIV or a weakened immune system increases your risks.

Pregnancy. Women who have had more than three full-term pregnancies or a first pregnancy before age seventeen are at increased risk for cancer of the cervix.

Oral contraceptives. Some studies have found a slightly increased risk of cervical cancer in those women who take the pill. It is unclear whether this is because oral contraceptives cause changes in the cells of the cervix that make them more susceptible to HPV infection, or whether women who take the pill are more likely to have unprotected sex and thus contract HPV. Regardless of the reason, the risk returns to normal after a woman stops taking the pill.

Symptoms

- Bleeding or spotting after sex
- Unusual vaginal discharge
- Pelvic pain
- Pain during sex

Screening

Pap smears screen for cervical cancer by sampling cells on and inside the cervix. If your Pap smear is abnormal, your doctor should be able to tell you precisely what type of abnormality it is and what it means. Cervical cancer usually takes ten to twenty years to develop, and cells go through progression from normal to slightly abnormal to precancerous to cancerous. Depending on the type of abnormality in your Pap smear, there will be clear guidelines for you to follow. Also, ask your doctor if he or she can test you specifically for HPV types 16 and 18. These types of HPV are known as high-risk subtypes and are associated with a higher risk of cervical cancer.

Prevention

In general, prevention of cervical cancer is simple: Practice safe sex, limit your number of sexual partners, don't smoke, and see your gynecologist regularly. Young women today can receive vaccinations against cervical cancer. However, these vaccines are not approved for women older than twenty-six. By age fifty, more than half of women have been exposed to HPV, and most do not get cervical cancer.

Stay Tuned

The world of cancer is changing as I write. Science and technology are improving the ways we diagnose and treat cancers of all types. Vaccines to prevent and treat cancer, personalized therapy, DNA "fingerprints" that indicate the presence of cancer, and improved genetic testing are being developed right now. Scientists are also learning more about the causes of cancer every day.

 DID YOU KNOW?
There may be a link between
sugar and cancer.

One exciting area of cancer research centers on sugar. When we eat sugar, high levels of insulin are released. Some scientists believe insulin works as a growth factor to stimulate tumors. If insulin is involved in making cancer cells grow, then blocking insulin's actions on cells some-how may turn out to be effective in treating cancer, too.[22]

While it's an exciting time for cancer research, your best defense against getting cancer is to live a healthy lifestyle. No matter how much treatments improve, your goal is to reduce your risk of getting cancer in the first place by committing to healthy habits that will keep your body beautiful, strong, and healthy.

Epilogue

Your Body Beautiful for Life

n this book, I've shared with you the best, most up-to-date research that medicine can offer on the science of staying beautiful, inside and out. Today, for the first time in history, we understand that the thirties and forties are not a time to coast, healthwise: They're the make-or-break decades for lifetime health. If you choose *right now* to make the effort, find the time, and commit to building healthy habits in the areas of eating, exercise, beauty, stress, and sex, you'll be choosing a path that leads to lifetime beauty, inside and out.

But this isn't a short-term program or a set-it-and-forget-it plan that you'll never change. Science is an evolving field, and breakthroughs will be part of our future. This book is not the last word on women's health issues, but the start of a lifelong dialogue. It reflects what I would tell you, doctor to patient and woman to woman, not just about medical facts, but about a lifelong approach to caring for your health.

As your life changes over the years—as you have kids or don't, as your career ebbs and flows, as you leave or reenter the dating pool, as your metabolism changes—you'll find you need to adjust old habits or develop new ones. My greatest hope is that this book does more than help you build the specific set of healthy habits that I describe here. I hope you've learned that you can create your own habits anytime you need to, or anytime new research sheds light on our understanding of health, fitness, and disease prevention.

In short, I hope this book helped you discover that you have it in you to change, to commit, to create a healthy, beautiful life for decades to come. I'll say it just one more time, as my parting thought to you: It's *your* body, Beautiful. Only you can keep it that way.

ACKNOWLEDGMENTS

As a physician, I really do think every body is a beautiful body. The understanding and appreciation of the mysteries, capacities, and abilities of the human body are what inspired me to become a doctor. As a specialist in women's health, I chose to dedicate my professional life to helping women find and maintain the best physical and mental condition possible. I was inspired to follow this path after watching my own ob-gyn, Dr. Ben Pascario, and his style of caring for me for nearly thirty years. I felt that he was my partner in health, that he knew me as a person, first as a teenager and then as an adult woman, and had my best interests, both physical and emotional, at heart. He not only helped me bring my own babies into the world, but also trained me as a surgeon in the operating room, and having been both his patient and his student as well as his friend has been one of the greatest gifts in my life. When I started my career as a doctor in 2000, I decided that I wanted to have the same impact on my patients and students that Dr. Pascario has had on me.

This type of partnership in health and wellness between a doctor and a patient is at the heart of the inspiration behind this book. In my medical career, I saw, unfortunately, all too often that women were often put on "autopilot" in terms of their mental and physical condition between the years of thirty and fifty, and I believe this represents a missed opportunity in terms of well-being. The years following the last labor and delivery contraction and before the first hot flash should be among the best of a woman's life! And in helping me to get this message out to women everywhere, I want to acknowledge the many people whose assistance made this book possible.

Forever in my mind and heart will be the incredible teachers I had the privilege of learning from during my medical training. From Dr. William Burke, who inspired me to pursue a the specialty of ob-gyn when I was a medical student at Columbia University, to Dr. Lisa Anderson, Dr. Edward Jew, Dr. Jacques Moritz, and Dr. Oded Langer, among others, these physicians taught me specifics about being a doctor that I will never forget. For believing that women need and deserve state-of-the-art information conveyed in an easy-to-relate-to manner, my literary agent, David Hale Smith, continues to be a champion of all issues regarding women and girls. My editor, Lucia Watson, and her team at Penguin show similar devotion to this important cause, and my collaborator, Christine Rojo, and I are about as in sync as two working moms who live three thousand miles away from each other can be! My talent agent, Kenneth Slotnick, and his team at William Morris Endeavor Entertainment have been enormously supportive in helping to bring the important platform of women's health to the forefront of media coverage.

In terms of the medical issues that I felt were so critical to include in this book, I could not have succeeded in providing this level of specific information without the professional assistance of my cadre of medical experts: Dr. Robert Ashton, thoracic surgeon and my husband; Dr. Oscar Garfein, cardiologist and my father; Dr. Evan Garfein, plastic surgeon and my brother; Dr. Jeffrey Rapaport, New Jersey dermatologist; and Dr. Patricia Desalvo, New Jersey dentist. For his support, continued friendship, and dedication to women's health, Dr. Mehmet Oz has my deepest respect and gratitude. My office staff, Carole Gittleman and Ana Olivera, have been invaluable sources of assistance and share my dedication to providing the highest caliber of health care to my patients of all ages. My friends and patients, such as Kathy Leventhal, Lynne Klatskin, and numerous others, have offered great insights into the concerns of women and the information that is so important to the patient during a

ACKNOWLEDGMENTS

doctor-patient encounter. And for always being there for a quick reality check or girlfriends' time-out, my friends Barbara Fedida, Dora Smagler, and Lisa Oz have my greatest love and appreciation.

The practical issues of completing this work could not have been possible without the stylistic assistance of my dream team: beautiful wardrobe supplied by Hamrah's, the brilliant work of makeup artist and hair stylist Dora Smagler, and the talented eye of famed photographer Michael Benabib.

Last, but perhaps most important, I want to thank my family. My mother, retired R.N. Dorothy Garfein; my father, Dr. Oscar Garfein; my children, Alex and Chloë; and my husband and best friend, Dr. Robert Ashton, were patient, enthusiastic, critical (when necessary), and selfless in making it possible for me to spend so many hours writing this book. They understand my devotion to my patients and to women everywhere and share my hope that this book will make a meaningful difference in their lives, and help to make every body beautiful, from the inside out.

NOTES

The Make-or-Break Years
1. Lally, Phillippa, et al., "How Are Habits Formed? Modelling Habit Formation in the Real World," *European Journal of Social Psychology* 40, no. 6 (2010): 998–1009.

1. The Five-Day/Two-Day Plan
1. Repinski, Karyn, "Face Facts: Too Much Sugar Causes Wrinkles," *Prevention* (October 2007).
2. WebMD, "Calories in Drinks and Popular Beverages," www.webmd.com/community/healthy-weight-8/calorie-chart.htm.
3. National Heart, Lung and Blood Institute, "Assessing Your Weight and Health Risk," http://www.nhlbi.nih.gov/health/public/heart/obesity/lose_wt/risk.htm.
4. Black, Rosemary, "Being Too Thin Will Age Your Face," *New York Daily News*, March 30, 2009.
5. Volkow, N. D., G. J. Wang, et al. "'Nonhedonic' Food Motivation in Humans Involves Dopamine in the Dorsal Striatum and Methylphenidate Amplifies This Effect," *Synapse* 44, no. 3 (2002): 175–80.
6. Gearhardt, A. N., et al., "Preliminary Validation of the Yale Food Addiction Scale," *Appetite* 52, no. 2 (2009): 430–36.
7. "Vegetarianism in America," *Vegetarian Times*, 2008, http://www.vegetariantimes.com/features/archive_of_editorial/667.
8. American Dietetic Association, 2003, http://www.eatright.org.

2. Sleek, Strong, Sexy
1. Werner, Christian, et al., "Beneficial Effects of Long-term Endurance Exercise on Leukocyte Telomere Biology," *Circulation* (November 2009): S492.
2. Boyles, Salynn, "Molecular Proof: Exercise Keeps You Young," *WebMD Health News*, December 1, 2009, http://www.webmd.com/fitness-exercise/news/20091201/molecular-proof-exercise-keeps-you-young.
3. Jarat, Peter, "A Healthy Mix of Rest and Motion," *The New York Times*, May 3, 2007.
4. Gibala, Martin, et al., "Short-term Sprint Interval versus Traditional Endurance Training: Similar Initial Adaptations in Human Skeletal Muscle and Exercise Performance," *Journal of Physiology* 575, no. 3 (2006): 901–11.
5. "Fountain of Youth in Your Muscles? Researchers Uncover Muscle-Stem Cell Mechanism in Aging," *Science Daily*, December 2, 2010.

6. Murray, F., "Weight Management: The Key to Disease Prevention," *Better Nutrition for Today's Living* 56, no. 7 (1994): 44.
7. Mayo Clinic, "Exercise: Seven Benefits of Regular Physical Activity," http://www.mayo clinic.com/health/exercise/HQ01676.

3. Secrets for Skin, Hair, and Beauty

1. Axelsson, J., et al., "Beauty Sleep: Experimental Study on the Perceived Health and Attractiveness of Sleep Deprived People," *British Medical Journal* (December 2010): 341.
2. The National Sleep Foundation, "How Much Sleep Do We Really Need?" www.sleepfoun dation.org/ /article/how-sleep-works/how-much-sleep-do-we-really-need.
3. Campbell, S. S., and P. J. Murphy, "The Nature of Spontaneous Sleep Across Adulthood," *Journal of Sleep Research* 16, no. 1 (March 2007): 24–32.
4. National Heart Lung and Blood Institute, National Institutes of Health, "Insomnia," Disease and Conditions Index, http://www.nhlbi.nih.gov/health/dci/Diseases/inso/inso_all .html.
5. National Sleep Foundation, "Women and Sleep," http://www.sleepfoundation.org/arti cle/sleep-topics/women-and-sleep.
6. Perricone, Dr. Nicholas, *The Perricone Prescription* (New York: William Morrow, 2002).
7. Fields, K., et al., "Bioactive Peptides," *Journal of Cosmetic Dermatology* 8 (2009): 8–13.
8. American Society for Aesthetic Plastic Surgery, "Highlights of the 2010 ASAPS Statistics on Cosmetic Surgery," http://www.surgery.org/sites/default/files/2010-quickfacts_0 .pdf.

4. Happiness Habits

1. Lehrer, Jonah, "Under Pressure: The Search for a Stress Vaccine," *Wired* (July 2010).
2. Pennebaker, James, "Writing About Emotional Experiences as a Therapeutic Process," *Psychological Science* 8, no. 3 (May 1, 1997): 162–66.
3. Ramirez, Gerardo, and Sian L. Beilock, "Writing About Testing Worries Boosts Exam Performance in the Classroom," *Science* 331, no. 6014 (January 14, 2011): 211–13.
4. Smalley, Susan, and Diana Winston, *Fully Present: The Science, Art and Practice of Meditation* (Cambridge, Mass.: Da Capo, 2010).
5. Taylor, S. E., L. C. Klein, B. P. Lewis, T. L. Gruenewald, R. A. R. Gurung, and J. A. Updegraff, "Female Responses to Stress: Tend and Befriend, Not Fight or Flight," *Psychological Review* 107, no. 3 (2000): 41–429.
6. Monti, D., C. Peterson, E. Shakin Kunkel, W. Hauck, E. Pequignot, et al., "A Randomized, Controlled Trial of Mindfulness-Based Art Therapy (MBAT) for Women with Cancer," *Psycho-Oncology* 15, no. 5 (2006): 363–73.
7. Wang, Jiongjiong, et al., "Gender Differences in Neural Response to Psychological Stress," *Social, Cognitive and Affective Neuroscience* 2, no. 3 (September 2007), http://www.ncbi .nlm.nih.gov/pmc/articles/PMC1974871/.

5. Prescription for Better Sex

1. American Psychiatric Association, *DSM-IV*, text rev. (Washington, D.C.: APA, 2000).
2. Kerner, Ian, "Six Health Benefits of Sex," *Huffington Post*, February 2, 2011.
3. Parker-Pope, Tara, "Viagra and Women," The *New York Times*, July 23, 2008.
4. Labrie, F., D. Archer, et al., "Effect of Intravaginal Dehydroepiandrosterone on Libido and Sexual Dysfunction in Postmenopausal Women," *Menopause* 16, no. 5 (2009): 923–31.

6. Sexual Health Makeover

1. Centers for Disease Control and Prevention, "Genital Herpes Fact Sheet," http://www.cdc.gov/std/Herpes/STDFact-Herpes.htm.

2. Cherpes, Thomas L., Leslie A. Meyne, and Sharon L. Hillier, "Cunnilingus and Vaginal Intercourse Are Risk Factors for Herpes Simplex Virus Type 1 Acquisition in Women," *Sexually Transmitted Diseases* 32 (February 2005): 84–89.

7. Great Expectations

1. Centers for Disease Control, National Center for Health Statistics, National Vital Statistics System, "Cohort Fertility Statistics for All Women, 1960–2010," http://www.cdc.gov/nchs/nvss/cohort_fertility_tables.htm.

2. Trolice, M. P., "The State of ART," *Contemporary OB/GYN* (2010): 47–50.

3. Carpenter, M. W., and D. R. Coustan, "Criteria for Screening Tests for Gestational Diabetes," *American Journal of Obstetric Gynecology* 144 (1982): 768–73.

4. American College of Obstetrics and Gynecology, Committee on Obstetric Practice, "ACOG Committee Opinion No. 435: Postpartum Screening for Abnormal Glucose Tolerance in Women Who Had Gestational Diabetes Mellitus," *Obstetric Gynecology* 113, no. 6 (2009): 1419–21.

5. Lydon-Rochelle, M., et al., "Risk of Uterine Rupture During Labor Among Women with a Prior Cesarean Delivery," *New England Journal of Medicine* 345 (2001): 3–8.

6. "New Breastfeeding Study Shows Most Moms Quit Early," *Science Daily*, August 12, 2008.

7. Lucas, A., "Breast Milk and Subsequent Intelligence Quotient in Children Born Preterm," *The Lancet* 339 (1992): 261–62.

8. Hormones

1. Liu, J. H., and M. L. Gass, *Management of the Perimenopause* (New York: McGraw-Hill, 2006).

2. Bluming, A. Z., et al., "Hormone Replacement Therapy: Real Concerns and False Alarms," *Cancer* 15, no. 2 (March/April 2009).

3. LaCroix, A. Z., et al., "Health Outcomes After Stopping Conjugated Equine Estrogens Among Post-Menopausal Women with Prior Hysterectomy," *Journal of the American Medical Association* (April 2011): 1305–14.

4. Rosenthal, M. S., "Bioidentical Hormones: Ethics and Misinformed Consent," *Female Patient* 34 (August 2009): 28–31.

5. Lokkegaard, E., A. H. Andreasen, A. K. Jacobsen, et al., "Hormone Therapy and Risk of Myocardial Infarction: A National Registry Study," *European Heart Journal* 29, no. 21 (2008): 2660–68.

6. Knutson, Mary Christine, "Facts and Fallacies of Menopause and Hormone Therapy," *Medscape Education*, December 12, 2003.

7. Van Die, M. D., et al., "Vitex Agnus-Castus in the Treatment of Menopause-Related Complaints," *Journal of Alternative and Complementary Medicine* 15, no. 8 (2009): 853–62.

9. Beauty and the Breast

1. American Society for Aesthetic Plastic Surgery, "Top Five Surgical and Nonsurgical Procedures in 2010," http://www.surgery.org/sites/default/files/2010-top5.pdf.

2. Ibid.

3. American Cancer Society, "Mammograms and Other Breast Imaging Procedures," www.cancer.org.

4. Li, C., et al., "Alcohol Consumption and Risk of Postmenopausal Breast Cancer by Sub-type: The Women's Health Initiative Observational Study," *Journal of the National Cancer Institute* 102, no. 18 (2010): 1422–31.
5. Harvie, M., et al. "Association of Gain and Loss of Weight Before and After Menopause with Risk of Postmenopausal Breast Cancer in the Iowa Women's Health Study," *Cancer Epidemiology, Biomarkers, & Prevention* 14, no. 3 (March 2005): 656–61.
6. Chlebowski, R. T., et al., "Dietary Fat Reduction and Breast Cancer Outcome: Interim Efficacy Results from the Women's Intervention Nutrition Study," *Journal of the National Cancer Institute* 98, no. 24 (2006): 1767–76.
7. American Cancer Society, "Breast Cancer Overview," www.cancer.org.
8. Lin, J., "Intakes of Calcium and Vitamin D and Breast Cancer Risk in Women," *Archives of Internal Medicine* 10, no. 17 (May 28, 2007): 1050–59.
9. Goodwin P. J., et al., "Prognostic Effects of 25-hydroxyvitamin D Levels in Early Breast Cancer," *Journal of Clinical Oncology* 27 (2009): 3757–63.
10. Lin, J., "Intakes of Calcium and Vitamin D," 1052.
11. Steube, A., et al., "Lactation and Incidence of Premenopausal Breast Cancer," *Archives of Internal Medicine* 169, no. 15 (August 10, 2009): 1364–71.

10. The Heart of the Matter

1. Belkin, Douglas, "Not Many Americans Born with Blue Eyes," *San Diego Union-Tribune*, October 22, 2006.
2. United States Census Bureau, "Educational Attainment in the United States 2010, Table 1: Educational Attainment of Population 18 and Over, by Age, Sex, Race, and Hispanic Origin," http://www.census.gov.
3. Gallup News Service, "About One in Four Americans Can Hold a Conversation in a Second Language," April 6, 2001.
4. Mosca, L., et al., "Tracking Women's Awareness of Heart Disease: An American Heart Association National Study," *Circulation* 109 (2004): 573–79.
5. American Academy of Periodontology, "Gum Disease Links to Heart Disease and Stroke," May 8, 2008, http://www.perio.org/consumer/mbc.heart.htm.
6. Lloyd-Jones, Donald M., et al., "Hypertension in Adults Across the Age Spectrum: Current Outcomes and Control in the Community," *Journal of the American Medical Association* 294, no. 4 (2005): 466–72.
7. Mosca, L., et al., "Effectiveness-Based Guidelines for the Prevention of Cardiovascular Disease in Women: 2011 Update," *Journal of the American College of Cardiology* 57 (2011): 1404–23.
8. Singh, J. P., J. C. Evans, D. Levy, et al., "Prevalence and Clinical Determinants of Mitral, Tricuspid, and Aortic Regurgitation (The Framingham Heart Study)," *American Journal of Cardiology* 83, no. 6 (March 15, 1999): 897–902.
9. Carpenter, A. J., et al., "Valvular Heart Disease in Women: The Surgical Perspective," *Journal of Thoracic and Cardiovascular Surgery* 127 (2004): 4–6.
10. Goland, S., K. Modi, F. Bitar, M. Janmohamed, J. M. Mirocha, L. S. Czer, et al., "Clinical Profile and Predictors of Complications in Peripartum Cardiomyopathy," *Journal of Cardiac Failure* 15, no. 8 (October 2009): 645–50.
11. Mehta, N. J., R. N. Mehta, and I. A. Khan, "Peripartum Cardiomyopathy: Clinical and Therapeutic Aspects," *Angiology* 52, no. 11 (November 2001): 759–62.
12. Bugiardini, R., O. Manfrini, C. Pizzi, F. Fontana, and G. Morgagni, "Endothelial Function Predicts Future Development of Coronary Artery Disease: A Study of Women with Chest Pain and Normal Coronary Angiograms," *Circulation* 109 (2004): 2518–23.

13. Mosca, L., et al., "AHA Guidelines, Effectiveness-Based Guidelines for the Prevention of Cardiovascular Disease in Women—2011 Update," *Circulation* 123 (2011): 1243–62.
14. Mieres, J. H., L. J. Shaw, A. Arai, et al., "Role of Noninvasive Testing in the Clinical Evaluation of Women with Suspected Coronary Artery Disease: Consensus Statement from the Cardiac Imaging Committee, Council on Clinical Cardiology, and the Cardiovascular Imaging and Intervention Committee, Council on Cardiovascular Radiology and Intervention, American Heart Association," *Circulation* 111 (2005): 682–96.

11. Boning Up

1. Bliue, D., N. Nguyen, V. Milch, T. Nguyen, J. Eisman, et al., "Mortality Risk Associated with Low-Trauma Osteoporotic Fracture and Subsequent Fracture in Men and Women," *Journal of the American Medical Association* 301, no. 5 (2009): 513–21.
2. Ibid.
3. Ibid.
4. Ibid.
5. National Institutes of Health, U.S. Department of Health and Human Services, "Bone Health and Osteoporosis: A Report of the Surgeon General," October 14, 2004, http://www.surgeongeneral.gov/library/bonehealth/content.html.
6. Ibid.
7. New, Susan, and Jean-Philippe Bonjour, eds., *Nutritional Aspects of Bone Health* (Cambridge: Royal Society of Chemistry, 2003): 440.
8. Bredella, M., "Effects of Visceral Obesity on Bone Health," paper presented at RSNA 2010: The 96th Annual Conference of the Radiological Society of North America, Chicago, November 30, 2010, http://rsna2010.org/program/event_display.cfm?em_id-9006863.
9. Taylor, Rebecca Buffum, "Osteoporosis and Men," WebMD, http://www.webmd.com/osteoporosis/living-with-osteoporosis-7/male-men.
10. Ibid.
11. FDA Patient Safety News, "FDA Update on Femur Fracture Risk with Bisphosphonates," January 2011, http://www.fda.gov/psn/transcript.cfm?show=106.

12. On the Attack

1. American Cancer Society, *Cancer Facts & Figures 2010* (Atlanta: American Cancer Society, 2010).
2. Doheny, Kathleen, "Fifteen Cancer Symptoms Women Ignore," WebMD, http://www.webmd.com/cancer/features/15-cancer-symptoms-women-ignore.
3. National Cancer Lung Partnership, "Lung Cancer Facts," http://www.nationallungcancerpartnership.org/lung-cancer-info/lung-cancer-facts.
4. Office of the Surgeon General, U.S. Department of Health and Human Services, "The Health Consequences of Involuntary Exposure to Tobacco Smoke: A Report of the Surgeon General," June 27, 2006, http://www.surgeongeneral.gov/library/secondhandsmoke/.
5. Rabin, R. C., "A New Cigarette Hazard: Thirdhand Smoke," *The New York Times*, June 2, 2009.
6. The National Cancer Institute, "Lung Cancer Prevention," http://www.cancer.gov/cancertopics/pdq/prevention/lung/Patient/page3.
7. Bourzac, K., "Lung Cancer Breathalyzer," *Technology Review* (March 2, 2007).
8. American Cancer Society, "Colorectal Cancer Overview," 2011, http://www.cancer.org/Cancer/ColonandRectumCancer/OverviewGuide/colorectal-cancer-overview-survival-rates.
9. Runowicz, Carolyn D., Sheldon H. Cherry, et al., *The Answer to Cancer* (Emmaus, PA: Rodale, 2004): 151–58.

10. Ibid.
11. Rothwell, P. M., et al., "Long-term Effects of Aspirin on Colorectal Cancer Incidence and Mortality: Twenty-Year Follow-up of Five Randomized Trials," *The Lancet* 376, no. 9754 (2010): 1741–50.
12. American Cancer Society, "Key Statistics About Thyroid Cancer," June 29, 2011, http://www.cancer.org/Cancer/ThyroidCancer/DetailedGuide/thyroid-cancer-key-statistics.
13. Wagner, J. D., M.S. Gordon, T. Y. Chuang, and J. J. Coleman III, "Current Therapy of Cutaneous Melanoma," *Plastic and Reconstructive Surgery* 105 (2001): 1774–99.
14. Runowicz, *The Answer to Cancer,* p. 153.
15. American Academy of Dermatology, "Indoor Tanning Tax Sends Strong Health Message: Indoor Tanning Is Unsafe," News release, June 30, 2011, http://www.aad.org/stories-and-news/news-releases/indoor-tanning-tax-sends-strong-health-message-indoor-tanning-is-unsafe.
16. Ovarian Cancer National Alliance, "Statistics," http://www.ovariancancer.org/about-ovarian-cancer/statistics.
17. Ibid.
18. Pat, T., et al., "BRCA1 and BRCA2 Mutations Account for a Large Proportion of Ovarian Carcinoma Cases," *Cancer* 104, no. 12 (2005): 2807–16.
19. Runowicz, *The Answer to Cancer,* p. 165.
20. Ibid.
21. Emons, G., G. Fleckenstein, B. Hinney, A. Huschmand, and W. Heyl, "Hormonal Interactions in Endometrial Cancer," *Endocrine-Related Cancer* 7, no. 4 (2000): 227–42.
22. Taubes, G., "Is Sugar Toxic?" *The New York Times Magazine,* April 13, 2011.

INDEX